Joe's
$170,000
Broken Leg

Joe's
$170,000
Broken Leg

CHARLES PETER, MD

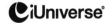iUniverse®

JOE'S $170,000 BROKEN LEG

iUniverse books may be ordered through booksellers or by contacting:

iUniverse
1663 Liberty Drive
Bloomington, IN 47403
www.iuniverse.com
1-800-Authors (1-800-288-4677)

ISBN: 978-1-5320-9450-7 (sc)
ISBN: 978-1-5320-9451-4 (e)

Library of Congress Control Number: 2020902066

Print information available on the last page.

iUniverse rev. date: 02/21/2020

Foreword

The insurance cartel, with their lackey lawyers, ruined our health-care system by driving the cost of liability (malpractice) insurance to a level inconsistent with the private practice of medicine.

The yearly cost of malpractice insurance in the nation is $56.5 billion, or 2.4 percent of the health-care cost. Defensive medicine costs dwarf this amount. Defensive medicine has morphed into a maximization of income by doctors and hospitals, the cost of which dwarfs the cost of defensive medicine.

The insurance cartel has convinced the masses that everyone should be compensated every step of the way on the inexorable march to the grave.

The cost of health care in the United States is about $1.7 trillion. So much of this is the result of paperwork, government regulations, fraud, and maximizing income (thievery) by doctors and hospitals that $300–400 billion easily could be cut from the $1.7 trillion without diminishing the quality of care. That would be $1,000 for every person in the country, which would be a great economic stimulus.

Our country is not a republic; it is a corporate oligarchy.

It is amazing that the insurance cartel was able to get its lobbyists, known in other parts of the country as "bagmen," to convince our lawmakers to pass a bill requiring everyone in the country to buy an insurance policy he or she did not need, did not want, and could not afford.

The insurance cartel fixed it so a person can buy health insurance from only two or three companies that are allowed to operate in a state.

We do not need a health-care bill, but we are going to get one as soon as the insurance cartel's lobbyists can write one and get the lawmakers to pass it. The upcoming health-care bill will better position the insurance oligarchs at the government trough and at the citizen's wallet.

One-payer government medicine will be administered by insurance companies. This is why the insurance cartel wrecked the private practice of medicine.

Medicaid in Texas has one payer. Years ago, Texas Medicaid was run by the National Heritage Insurance Company, owned by Ross Perot, who amassed a fortune of $4 billion. Later, Medicaid was administered by UnitedHealthcare, whose CEO had $1.7 billion in unexercised stock options. Turn the fat hogs out and the lean hogs in.

President Trump worries about manufacturing jobs leaving the country. It costs too much to manufacture anything in this country because of

- taxes,
- governmental regulations,

- lawyers,
- unions, and
- health care!

The government is unconcerned about the cost of health care because the government has no competition, can print money, and can't go broke.

The insurance cartel is unconcerned about the cost of health care because the higher the cost, the higher the premiums.

Hospitals are unconcerned about the cost of health care because the higher the bills, the more money they make.

Patients don't care about the cost because they think someone else is paying for it.

Corporations must control the cost of health care for which they are paying in order to compete in the marketplace. Patients who pay for health care directly would be interested in controlling the cost of health care. Health savings accounts might accomplish this.

Health care is not a widget; it is a product containing a large number of things and a large number of costs, many of which are designed to maximize income rather than to benefit the patient.

Over fifty years ago, when I first came to Houston, a family practitioner had a sixty- or sixty-three-year-old patient too young for Medicare—a mechanic with a hiatal hernia that caused his food to come up when he rolled under a car to work on it.

The patient had $500 to spend on an operation. As

a favor to the family practitioner, the small hospital took $350; I took the other $150.

With the family doctor as an assistant, we repaired the patient's hiatal hernia using a technique described by Mr. Belsey, a British surgeon with the title "Mister" instead of "Doctor"—a throwback to the barber surgeons who bled people as a method of treatment.

Mr. Belsey's operation involved opening the left chest and looking down on the esophagus where it entered the stomach. The stomach had slipped into the chest because the hole in the diaphragm through which the esophagus goes to join the stomach had enlarged, allowing the stomach to reside in the chest, removing the valve-like mechanism that the normal anatomy permits.

There is a right and a left vagus nerve running down either side of the esophagus, but at the level of the diaphragm, these are more like anterior and posterior vagus nerves.

Mr. Belsey's operation involved putting two rows of mattress sutures (sutures going in one way and back the opposite way and being tied) from the esophagus to the stomach. On top of this layer of sutures, a second layer, going in and out of the diaphragm, was put in, pulling the stomach below the diaphragm, where the stomach belongs. The two or three previously placed sutures in the diaphragm would then be tied, and the chest closed.

Today hiatal hernias are repaired through the abdomen by using a laparoscope to wrap the fundus of the stomach around the esophagus, restoring the valve-like mechanism that keeps food in the stomach.

Holes in the abdominal wall are not nearly as

debilitating as a thoracotomy and allow the patient to return to work sooner.

Some interests in the United States say calling surgeons "Mister" is as it should be, implying that surgeons are less than doctors.

Perhaps bleeding helped patients; if you are anemic, your body makes more red blood cells and possibly more white blood cells that fight infections. At that time there were no government grants to fund a double-blind study. Perhaps the placebo effect was in play with bleeding.

At this time, my malpractice premiums were $600; when I quit operating on people, the premiums approached $50,000. A neurosurgeon in Philadelphia was paying $350,000 a year; cardiac surgeons, $100,000; ob-gyns, very large sums; and a surgeon in Dade County (Miami), Florida, $90,000.

Today, a patient would have his or her hiatal hernia repaired with a laparoscope costing many thousands of dollars.

Exorbitant malpractice premiums affect not only the doctors but also the hospitals, drug companies, and medical device companies.

Joe, a diabetic living in a small town near a big city, left his business to go home and watch a baseball game on TV. On his way home, Joe became nauseated and dizzy; he ran his truck into a ditch, breaking his leg. The ambulance came, but Joe wanted his wife to take him home.

About twenty years ago, Joe's wife made him go to the doctor because he was not feeling well. Joe had a blood sugar of 400 mg/dl instead of 100 mg/dl. The complications of diabetes are reduced if one's blood sugar is well controlled. Joe controlled his blood sugar with missionary zeal; he was too zealous at times. Joe had had hypoglycemia (low blood sugar) on several occasions. This is what caused Joe's accident. If one's blood sugar is too low, one becomes dizzy, sweats, and may pass out or have a convulsion. Sugar is urgently needed at such times.

Diabetes is divided into two groups: type I, or insulin-dependent, diabetes; and type II diabetes, also known as non-insulin-dependent diabetes or adult-onset diabetes.

Type I diabetes is caused by a lack of insulin being produced by the islet cells in the pancreas. It is thought to be caused by the body's immune system destroying these cells, perhaps brought on by a viral infection. Babies can develop diabetes after a viral infection.

Type II diabetes accounts for 90 to 95 percent of diabetes and affects 25.8 million Americans, or 8.3 percent of the population. Type II diabetics have insulin, but it doesn't work well. Most, if not all, type II diabetics are overweight. If one's parent has diabetes, one has a 50 percent chance of developing diabetes; if both parents have diabetes, the chance is 100 percent. This is qualified by saying "If one lives long enough." What is long enough?

Today, a hemoglobin A1c test can determine how well the blood sugar of a diabetic has been controlled over the past several days.

When Joe's leg pain did not go away after two or three

days, he went to the emergency room at a large hospital in the nearby city. He had a broken leg—a fractured femur.

Nineteen days and $143,000 later, Joe was discharged. The $143,000 came from $7,526.31 charged per day, not including bills from his several doctors, outpatient physical therapy, and visits to his "pain doctor." Patients don't get an itemized bill unless they ask for one. The patient doesn't care what is on the bill, because insurance is paying for it.

Joe's hospital bill was as follows:

016	Pharmacy	13,887.00
019	Med/Surg Supplies	17,265.50
026	Laboratory	11,472.35
028	Radiology-Diagnostic	2,513.75
032	Operating Room Services	11,645.75
033	Anesthesia	6,328.25
035	Blood processing & storage	2,022.00
036	Imaging Services	908.00
038	Physical Therapy	3,114.00
042	Emergency Room	3,412.75
064	Post Anesthesia Care	1,981.25
066	EKG/ECG	697.98
088	Peripheral Vascular Service	2,251.00
151	Unknown	3,729.00
	Total Charges	103,546.35
	Bill from other pages	43,053.00

Room, board, and nursing services at $1,155.00 per day cost approximately $21,000. This included room, food, and twenty-four-hour-a-day nurses. This was about

$47 per hour. One nurse usually takes care of four or more patients. Also, there are ward clerks, nurses' aides, and orderlies. Much of the cost is for liability insurance and workers' compensation for employees. Much of the nurses' time is spent charting or computing—perhaps more time than is spent with patients.

016   Pharmacy

Zofran—4 caps $540.00
A hospital sent out a memo asking the doctors to use cheaper antinausea drugs than Zofran, which costs $113. Zofran cost the hospital $13; the hospital charged $113. There were no Zofran caps when the above memo was sent out. Oral Zofran is especially good because it can be given to young children; phenothiazine and Phenergan can't.

Omeprazole $64.00
Four caps to lower stomach acid can be bought over the counter at any pharmacy. Larry the Cable Guy could have gotten a better deal.

Augmentin—antibiotic given in ER $90.50
Augmentin, penicillin with something added to it, was given to Joe in the emergency room. In 1936, Dr. Fleming in England left the tops off two plates, one growing bacteria and the other growing fungus. When some of the fungus blew over and killed the bacteria, penicillin

was discovered. Penicillin was truly a wonder drug. However, over the years, more and more bacteria became resistant to penicillin, requiring that penicillin be modified. Augmentin is such a modified drug. Without seeing the chart, one can only surmise what was being treated. Because Joe was a diabetic, the antibiotic was given for prophylaxis, perhaps.

Hydralazine injection $322.00

This was administered to lower blood pressure. Joe had high blood pressure.

Fluticasone nasal spray $356.00

This is a cortisone nose spray for allergic rhinitis (a stopped-up nose). Joe was charged for fluticasone on October 20, October 23, and October 25, 2010, for a total of $1,068. The dose is two puffs in each nostril daily—usually one puff after the first day. There are 120 puffs in each container. Four puffs a day for nineteen days is about 80 puffs. Joe was charged for 360 puffs, or about 280 puffs that he did not get. Joe had no history of allergies, but he was charged over $1,000 to unstop his nose. Maybe there was another indication.

Darbepoetin $1,835.00

Darbepoetin is a recombinant erythropoietin that is made by the kidneys to help make red blood cells. It is given to patients with end-stage kidney disease and anemia. Many of these patients are on dialysis. Increased hemoglobin levels usually don't occur until two to four weeks after treatment starts, which would have been after Joe had left the hospital. Blood clots are a side effect or complication of darbepoetin injection. Joe developed a clot in his arm vein even though he was receiving low-molecular-weight heparin. Most likely the clot in Joe's arm vein was caused by all the drugs infused in his arm vein rather than due to the darbepoetin.

Xenaderm—60 g ×2 $294.00
Xenaderm is an ointment to put on the sacrum to help prevent bedsores. Not only do bedsores generate a number of lawsuits, but in Florida, one might be put in jail for neglect of an old person if neglect is proven, and bedsores can serve as such proof.

Levofloxacin—antibiotic
Levofloxacin is a broad-spectrum quinolone-class drug. There may have been a question as to whether it might cause the rupture of Achilles tendons. This drug cannot be given to people less than eighteen years of age because of the effect on cartilage. The last epiphysis to close is in the shoulder blade, and it closes at about seventeen to eighteen years of age. The epiphysis is the end of the bone, where growth takes place. Levofloxacin

may cause aortic valve disease or cause one's Achilles tendon to rupture. It is recommended that an alternate be used if possible.

Cefepime—antibiotic
Cefepime is a fourth-generation cephalosporin. It kills staphylococcus and pseudomonas. Most antibiotics don't.

Vancomycin—antibiotic
Vancomycin kills gram-positive bacteria. Bacteria are classified as cocci and rods and as gram positive (black) and gram negative (red). This relates to the color of the bacteria when stained with a gram stain. The cocci (round dots) are usually gram positive and reside on the skin and in the upper respiratory tract. The gonococcus is an exception; it is two round dots mashed together, thus a diplococcus. If one sees intracellular (in-cell) gram-negative diplococci, one is seeing gonorrhea. The rods are usually gram negative (red) and reside in the intestines. However, the genus Clostridium is gram positive (black) and includes tetanus, gas gangrene, and *Clostridium difficile*.

Today many of the staphylococci (which cause boils and skin infections) are resistant to most every antibiotic except vancomycin, which must be given parenterally, because it is not absorbed from the intestine. Vancomycin blood levels must be checked twice daily, at peak and trough levels. If the vancomycin level is too low, the drug is ineffective; if too high, the drug damages the kidneys. Now there is Zyvox, an oral drug that kills resistant staph, as does vancomycin. It costs several hundred dollars a pill. Oral vancomycin is used to treat *Clostridium difficile*, a gram-positive bacteria that normally lives in the colon. When antibiotics kill the bacteria in the colon, *Clostridium difficile* flourishes and causes ulcers and sometimes death. Tetanus and gas gangrene are caused by Clostridium-genus bacteria. Flagyl, taken by mouth, is also used to treat *Clostridium difficile*. Although probably not the best drug, resistance of staph and enterococci to vancomycin is prevented. Oral Flagyl also makes one nauseated after a few days. Those who say otherwise probably haven't taken Flagyl. *Clostridium difficile* infection can occur in elderly people (defined as someone fifteen years older than the doctor) who have not taken antibiotics. In years gone by, *Clostridium difficile* was treated by giving the patient a fecal enema. This was somewhat less than aesthetically pleasing to some. This was done to restock the colon with normal intestinal bacteria, restoring the colon's normal flora. *Clostridium difficile* infection is diagnosed by examining the stool for *Clostridium difficile* toxin titer. False negatives are not uncommon. Questran, which looks like ground-up birdseed, can be used when mixed with a liquid and taken by mouth to treat *Clostridium difficile* diarrhea as well as any other diarrhea. Questran binds bile and is especially useful for treating diarrhea following a cholecystectomy.

If there is a chance that the diarrhea is caused by *Clostridium difficile*, one should not use Imodium, Lomotil, or other drugs that stop peristalsis, because if the intestinal contents aren't evacuated, the germs will just sit there and eat on one another.

Cefazolin—cephalosporin
One of the first drugs of its class, Cefazolin is good for gram-positive bacteria but has been replaced in most cases.

Nystatin—oral antifungal
When antibiotics kill all the bacteria, fungus will grow.

Bacitracin $153.00
Bacitracin is an antibiotic used to irrigate surgical wounds, usually too toxic to take parenterally.

Warfarin $294.00
Warfarin is an oral anticoagulant that blocks vitamin K, which is necessary for blood clotting. Because Joe had a clot in his arm vein, he was given anticoagulants after he left the hospital. When one

takes warfarin, it is necessary to have one's blood checked twice a week. Several things interfere with warfarin. Spinach is one of them. Warfarin is used as rat poison; it causes the rats to bleed to death.

Nifedipine $33.00

Nifedipine lowers blood pressure by blocking calcium from entering the cell.

Carvedilol $16.00

Carvedilol is an alpha and beta blocker used for lowering blood pressure. Epinephrine (Adrenalin) is an alpha and beta body chemical.

Labetalol $29.00

Labetalol is a beta blocker for lowering blood pressure; it decreases the force of contraction of the heart. Other beta blockers might be used primarily to slow the heart rate and also lower blood pressure.

The adrenal glands lie atop the kidneys. The cortex of the gland produces cortisone, and the medulla, or the rest of the gland, produces epinephrine (80 percent)—better known by its trade name, Adrenalin—which acts on the heart as well as on the blood vessels and bronchi (windpipes), and norepinephrine (20 percent), which acts primarily on blood vessels.

Asthma is a disease of constriction of the small airways in the lungs. Beta drugs dilate these airways; therefore, one must be careful when giving a beta blocker to an asthmatic.

Most of Joe's blood pressure drugs were beta blockers.

Ophthalmic lubricant—3.5 grams $29.50
This is grease put in the eyes during anesthesia to prevent the eyeballs from drying.

Fentanyl—anesthesia drug $9.00
Fentanyl is a very powerful narcotic used in general anesthesia.

Vecuronium—anesthesia drug, muscle $33.00
relaxant

Rocuronium—anesthesia drug, muscle $99.00
relaxant
Curare was the first muscle relaxant. The natives put it on their darts and shot monkeys in the trees. Synthetic muscle relaxants have been developed. Anectine causes muscle fasciculation before complete relaxation, causing potassium to leave the cell and increasing the serum potassium. The potassium in the serum may be 4, but it may be 40 in the cell. A high potassium level will stop the heart; therefore, a patient with a high potassium level should be relaxed with a drug that does not cause fasciculation.

Propofol

Propofol, which looks like milk, is used in anesthesia to rapidly put the patient to sleep before injecting muscle relaxants, powerful narcotics, and other drugs. Propofol was at the center of the Michael Jackson death trial that lasted for weeks. Michael Jackson was kept sleeping with a constant infusion of propofol. An autopsy showed that Michael Jackson had a lethal propofol level. Propofol is rapidly metabolized by the liver, and a single injection won't keep a patient asleep very long. It is unknown how long Michael Jackson was dead while the propofol was still dripping into his vein but not being metabolized by his liver because he was dead. When the emergency crew arrived and started chest compressions, the propofol that had dripped into the arm was circulated throughout the body. This would give a higher postmortem propofol level than the antemortem propofol level. From the media accounts, this was not brought up at Dr. Murray's trial. Dr. Murray was convicted and put in jail. When "they" decide to put you in jail, "they" put you in jail. There are more Michael Jackson voters than there are Dr. Murray voters. The judge might have been elected.

Epinephrine—drug to increase blood pressure
Apparently Joe developed low blood pressure during the operation.

019   Medical/surgical supplies

Blood administration sets	$241.50

Joe lost three to four pints of blood into his leg from the fracture, plus some from the operation.

Bandage—Coban self-adherent	$18.50
Cuff—VenaFlow disposable	$148.00
Guidewire Gamma	$511.00
Drill bit, Synthes, quick coupling (2)	$775.00

They probably needed to drill a hole in the top of the hip bone to put a rod down.

Imp screw, Skyline	$1,378.00
Imp screw, locking	$2,174.00
Ace bandage	$24.50
Dressing, Xeroform, large	$8.00
Imp screw, trochanteric fixation	$3,085.00
ESV pencil, Volloflab	$39.00
Imp Fix Nail Conn Trach Ti	$8,391.00
Rod, reaming, with ball tip, 950 mm	$317.00
Blood administration set	$80.50
	$17,265.50

This operation involved putting a titanium rod down the hole in the femur across the fracture to stabilize it, allowing the bone to heal. The above supplies are drill bits that were used to put a hole in the hip bone through which the rod was put.

Complaints caused the removal of a tax on medical devices to help fund Obamacare; otherwise the $17,265.50, would have been even higher.

026   Laboratory

Drug screen, single drug class $36.00
     This screen was levels of vancomycin.

Complete blood count $116.00
     A machine measures the number of red and white blood cells; perhaps platelets, which cause blood clotting, and hemoglobin, which transports oxygen. A family doctor can draw blood in his office and put the blood in a box on his door. A commercial laboratory will pick up the blood and fax the results to the doctor's office the next morning—all for five dollars. Of course, the doctor will charge for drawing the blood.

Coombs indirect $184.00
Coombs direct $80.00

     Coombs tests measure antibodies made by the immune system. The antibodies are stuck on the red blood cells. The indirect Coombs test uses serum; the direct Coombs test uses red blood cells. These tests were done because Joe got a blood transfusion. The test is used to cross-match the blood.

Blood has an A antigen and a B antigen, A&B or O, and it can be Rh positive or Rh negative. Type O Rh-negative blood should be able to be given to type A and B, Rh-positive patients. All blood transfusions are cross-matched with the recipient. Rh is named after the rhesus monkey, which was used to discover it.

Coombs tests are used in Rh-negative women who have had an Rh-positive baby because the father was Rh positive. If the Rh-negative mother has an Rh-positive baby, a miscarriage, an abortion, or an ectopic pregnancy, she needs to be given RhoGAM, an immunoglobulin, to prevent the formation of antibodies against the Rh factor, because if she gets pregnant again and has an Rh-positive baby, her Rh-positive antibodies from her previous pregnancy will attack the blood cells of the baby that she is carrying, causing a large problem for the fetus.

Rh-negative women should be given RhoGAM if they have had a miscarriage or an ectopic pregnancy. It is possible for a woman to have a miscarriage and think it a late or abnormal period.

What about our egalitarian army putting Rh-negative females into combat? Will the army use only Rh-positive blood, as was done in the Korean War? I don't know what kind of blood was used in Vietnam and Iraq. Four thousand have been killed in Iraq, thirty-five thousand in Vietnam, fifty-eight thousand in Korea, or vice versa, nineteen thousand and fifty thousand wounded in the Battle of the Bulge. Today, perhaps blood can be cross-matched. If not, will Rh-negative women be given RhoGAM to protect their future fetuses? Will it be enough RhoGAM if they have multiple transfusions? We are not all equal.

O is the most common blood type; Rh-positive is the most common Rh type. AB-negative is the rarest blood type. Because many people were trying to kill him, General de Gaulle, whose blood type was AB-negative, carried six bottles of AB-negative blood with him when he traveled. When visiting England, the general stored his blood in Lady Macmillan's refrigerator, causing the prime minister's wife extreme displeasure.

Theoretically, type O-negative blood could be transfused into anyone. Because Rh-negative blood is much less common than Rh-positive blood, during the Korean War, only O positive blood with a low Rh titer was used, eliminating cross-matching errors and shortages of certain types of blood. Plasma can be frozen; blood can't. Blood cells survive 120 days or less. The potassium level in the serum is about 4; in cells the potassium level is about 40. When many of the blood cells rupture, the potassium increases. Blood for transfusion can't be stored for 120 days.

Blood transfusions may not present a problem for those female combatants who never have been nor ever will be exposed to pregnancy unless it is by their savage captors.

Why are so many women attracted to women and so many men attracted to men? Could it be bisphenol-A (BPA), a hormone disrupter that affects both estrogens and androgens, which is used to make plastic bottles, food wrappers, pipe liners, and can liners? One study showed that mothers with high bisphenol-A levels had masculine daughters. Could a not-so-high bisphenol level in the mother produce a normal-appearing child with an alternate sexual preference?

The government has declared bisphenol-A safe, but the government has banned the use of bisphenol-A in making baby bottles. Might not the fetus be exposed to bisphenol-A if Mom sits around all day drinking water from a plastic bottle? A study could be done determining the bisphenol-A level in the mother's blood at birth as well as in the baby's umbilical cord blood.

How does one know what sexual orientation the baby will have? A pediatrician observed in a newborn nursery that newborn male babies' hands made fists and that newborn female babies' hands were open. Furthermore, the pediatrician noted that if a male baby's hands were open, he would have feminine tendencies, and if a female baby's hands made a fist, she would be masculine. This could be correlated with the bisphenol-A level in the umbilical cord blood at birth.

Yearly, 3.6 million tons, or 8 billion pounds, of bisphenol-A are produced, providing much money with which to hire lobbyists.

Niccolo Machiavelli, a Florentine public servant, attributed the fall the Roman Empire to their using Goths as mercenaries; others attributed the fall the Roman Empire to Attila the Hun; and still others attributed Rome's fall to their use of lead pipes, which gave the people lead poisoning and impaired their thinking.

Today will our empires fall because of our use of pipes made of bisphenol-A instead of lead, causing a decline of population because all the women are interested in women and all the men are interested in men?

Thromboplastin time test $144.00
> This test is used to check the anticoagulant effect of heparin.

Prothrombin time test $118.00
> This test warfarin (Coumadin). Several esoteric lab tests were done. Something must have caught the eye of a subspecialist. "If all that you have is a hammer, everything looks like a nail."

Parathyroid hormone intact test $525.25
> The parathyroid hormone regulates calcium in the blood. The calcium regulates the phosphorous

somewhat. When the calcium is elevated, the phosphorous is depressed.

The parathyroid glands are small glands, tan in color and about the size of one-half of a small green pea, located and attached to the underside of the upper and lower part of each side of the thyroid gland. Sometimes one of these glands can be in the chest. One must take care of these small glands when doing a thyroidectomy. A tumor or hyperplasia causes a high serum calcium, which may result in kidney stones. The calcium comes out of the bones.

Lipid Panel, October 21, 2010 $224.00

Lipid Panel, October 22, 2010 $224.00
I don't want to second-guess Joe's doctors, but I wonder why he needed two lipid panels to treat a broken leg.

Protein electrophoresis $103.75
I don't know what they were looking for with this.

Bence-Jones protein electrophoresis $324.00
This is a measurement to determine whether Bence-Jones protein is present. This protein is seen in patients with multiple myeloma, a cancer of one of the bone marrow cells. Multiple myeloma can cause holes in the bones. One treatment is to

kill all the bone marrow with chemotherapy then transplant new marrow into the patient.

Basic metabolic panel—total calcium × 8 $302.00
    This is a panel of tests that Joe had for eight days. Most likely Joe was eating during this time.

028 Radiology diagnostic	$2,513.75
Initial chest and femur x-ray	$329.25
	$441.50
Pelvis	$341.50
Other portable chest x-rays	$329.00
031 CT scans	
CT abdomen with contrast	$2,899.00
CT pelvis with contrast	$2,888.00
CT cervical spine without contrast	$3,437.00
CT head, routine	$2,421.45

Joe was in a one-car accident. His truck ran into a ditch three or four days before he came to the hospital. He was never unconscious. Maybe there were signs and symptoms that demanded these CT scans. Maybe they were carried out in the interest of being thorough. Maybe it was defensive medicine. If the diagnosis of appendicitis is in doubt and one wants to order a CT scan, one has to order two CT scans, abdomen and pelvis, because the appendix is between the two scans and one scan might miss it.

    These charges do not include the charges for the radiologist's interpretations, which could be $600 apiece. As the country and western song laments, "Mothers, don't let your sons grow up to be cowboys." Mothers, have your sons be radiologists. It probably took the radiologist less than twenty minutes to read and dictate all these CT scans. Medicare, of course, won't pay nearly this much.

A CT scan supposedly increases one's chances of cancer to 1 in 500 over one's lifetime. Four CT scans, of course, would make that 4 in 500.

032 Operating room services—5 hours $13,254.25
It takes some time to put the patient to sleep, prep him, and drape him after positioning him on the operating table, as well as some time to awaken him and put on a bandage.

Operations taking one hour or less have one level of complications; three hours, more complications; and over five hours, even more complications. Joe's operation took between three and five hours. He was charged $101.00 for norepinephrine and epinephrine, vasopressers, to increase his blood pressure, suggesting that Joe had low blood pressure during his operation.

033 Anesthesia		$5,885.25
Suprano, per bottle		$443.00
	Total	$6,328.25

The charge for the operating room should cover the machine. The anesthesiologist usually sends his or her own bill.

035 Blood processing and storage $2,022.00
The blood is free, to avoid the implied warranty law, which states that that which is sold should not harm people. This avoids lawsuits for AIDS, hepatitis, mismatched blood, and so on. Blood banks charge for processing the blood and usually have a name such as "Blood Services of Mudville" (or wherever).

036 Imaging Services $908.00
These included x-rays and Doppler studies on Joe's extremities, looking for blood clots. Joe had a blood clot in his arm, probably from irritation caused by all the drugs infused.

038 Physical therapy $3,114.00
The itemized bill shows $7,229.75 for physical therapy for eight days and $7,978.50 for occupational therapy for eight days. Perhaps the hospital did not want $15,000 on the bill where it could be seen at a glance. This is about $2,000 a day for eight days.

Physical therapy involved getting Joe out of bed to walk—a job previously relegated to nurses and nurses' aides.

Occupational therapy involves strengthening patients to be able to feed themselves, brush their teeth, and wipe their behinds. On November 5, 2010, Joe spent one and a half hours in physical therapy and one and a half hours in occupational therapy.

042 Emergency room

Joe's case was not a real emergency, because his leg had been broken for three days. However, he needed a diagnosis to be admitted to the hospital; besides, he could not wait days for an appointment with an orthopedist. He had an indwelling catheter for $630.00 and two liters of intravenous fluids for $1,048.00.

064 Post-anesthesia care $1,981.25

This is for the recovery room where the patient awakens from anesthesia. It takes longer for the recoveries of some patients than for others. A patient who had a five-hour anesthetic may take longer to recover.

051 Peripheral vascular examination $3,729.50

This involves Doppler studies (ultrasounds) to check for clots in the leg and arm veins. Both legs were examined on October 15, 2010, and one leg was again examined on October 20, 2010.

Unknown $3,729.50

Most people would not want to pay a bill unless they knew what it was for. Apparently Uncle Sugar doesn't care. If a business or a corporation were responsible for this bill, the bill would have been examined more closely. If the patient thinks that someone else is paying the bill, he or she doesn't worry about it.

Hospitals

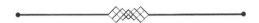

If one goes to a hospital emergency room, one can expect to be robbed. If one is admitted to a hospital and has no insurance, one can expect the same. Hospitals pad their bills and greatly discount the bill for Medicare, Medicaid, and insurance companies, but not for patients paying cash. This encourages people to buy insurance.

One-half of the personal bankruptcies were due to medical bills. Many had health insurance, or perhaps thought that they had health insurance but were denied by the insurance company for preexisting conditions or for other reasons. Some say that the high school dropouts at the insurance company get bonuses for denying claims.

The emergency room doctors at teaching hospitals are probably interns and residents. The for-profit hospitals' emergency room doctors most likely are furnished by a company. If the ER doctors don't overutilize, will the hospital CEO be displeased and get another group of ER doctors? The CEO might be replaced if the hospital doesn't make money. A hospital committee said that too many CT scans were being done in the ER. The next week, a patient with appendicitis was sent home. What is the answer? Better doctors.

A young man was beaten on the head with a bong. He did not need to go to a hospital, but the sheriff made him go to a hospital in an ambulance anyway. An ER doctor looked at him for about a minute, ordered an unnecessary CT scan of the head, discharged him, and sent him a bill for $700. The CT scan was $3,000, the radiologist charged $600 to read it, and the emergency room visit cost another $3,000.

A landscaper had a heart attack and went to a hospital emergency room. He had cardiac catheterization and stents placed. His total bill was $90,000. He had no health insurance. When he asked for a payment plan, he was refused and was told that the hospital wanted full payment now.

A forty-two-year-old respiratory technician went to a hospital emergency room because he had a kidney stone. He knew that he was passing a kidney stone because he had had this problem before. He was left in the hall and not put into a room. He was given no drugs, saw no doctor, passed the stone, was given a strainer to catch the stone, and was discharged. He had no insurance. His bill was $9,000. After he had paid about $4,000, he was told to pay up or he would be turned over to a collection agency, ruining his credit.

Most people can't pay cash for a car and need credit. These hospitals are stealing from and are fouling these people.

A patient had tonsil cancer with metastasis to a lymph

node in his neck. His dumb family doctor treated the lump for several months before the patient went to a cancer hospital in the city. He was supposed to die in six months, but three years later he was alive with radiation necrosis of his mandible. His insurance company paid $2–3 million. He paid $100,000 of his own money.

A woman had a hysterectomy for bleeding fibroids. Her hospital bill was $25,000. The insurance company paid $5,000, and she paid $500.

To put these charges in perspective, California pays twelve dollars for a Medicaid outpatient visit, and Texas eighteen dollars, soon to be reduced. The ER doctor pays a liability insurance premium. The doctor who sees Medicaid patients pays medical liability premiums, as well as office overhead (e.g., rent, phone, employees, worker's compensation insurance, and perhaps health insurance for his employees).

The governor of Florida, a former Hospital Corporation of America (HCA) executive who, according to newspaper articles, spent $50 million of his own money getting elected, said on one of his shows that we should have lower taxes in order for corporations to compete in world markets. If not a tax on business, what does he think health-care costs are, if companies with fifty employees have to offer their employees health insurance?

Another newspaper article told of a nephrologist in Florida who complained about HCA dialysis hospitals not giving the drugs that he ordered, among other things. One hospital was fined $800, and the nephrologist was not reappointed to the staff. This whopping fine really bothered this corporation that made over a billion dollars in one year.

The article also said that HCA had "aggressive billing," which, in my opinion, based on known facts, may or may not be a euphemism for stealing.

A patient entered a Hospital Corporation of America (HCA) hospital because air leaked from a diverticulum in his small amount of remaining colon. The patient spent two nights in the hospital; he was charged for one day. The patient was hooked up to telemetry, an electrocardiogram that comes across a screen at a nursing station, for twenty-four hours a day, even though the doctor didn't order it. The telemetry was discontinued when the patient pointed this out to his doctor.

Why do the doctors sign the orders for telemetry that they do not order? A month later, the doctor signed everything on the chart with his sticky on it; maybe HCA would not appoint him to the staff as a Florida nephrologist.

If telemetry costs $150 an hour, $1,800 a day, $657,000 a year, then just one patient each in 163 hospitals would be $107,091,000 over the course of a year. Fifty dollars an hour would be one-third of this amount.

HCA adds a technical anesthesia charge to each operation that requires a general anesthetic. The patient is charged for the drugs used and for the operating room. The anesthesiologist sends a separate bill. Most likely, some of the $500 is used to pay the nurse anesthetist, who is not allowed to charge. Five hundred dollars added to twenty operations a day at 163 hospitals, 250 days a year, is about $400 million.

According to a nurse at an HCA hospital, patients are charged to be rolled to and from the operating suite, as well as charged to wait in the holding area for their operations. Talk about "aggressive billing."

At some of the long-term-care hospitals, it is not known about HCA hospitals that when a tube is passed into the stomach (a nasogastric tube), to make sure that the tube is in the stomach and not coiled in the esophagus or in the lung, someone listens over the stomach with a stethoscope while air is squirted into the tube. A gurgling sound can be heard, assuring the listener that the tube is in the stomach. Also, the tube can be put under water to see if air is coming out, indicating that the tube is in the lung. This has worked well since nasogastric tubing was first used, but now an x-ray is taken to check the tube's position, requiring an x-ray technician, a radiologist to dictate a report, and a house doctor to look at the x-ray when the tube was placed.

Perhaps some of our foreign nurses are not competent enough to put nasogastric tubes in, or perhaps this is a new revenue stream. If a company or a corporation paid the hospital for the company's employees, this probably would not be allowed.

According to a newspaper ad, HCA was taken private by Bain Capital and two other like enterprises. Governor Romney did not tout HCA as one of Bain Capital's stellar successes.

Had Joe gone to a HCA hospital, his bill might have been more. Probably not; it appears that all hospitals practice "aggressive billing."

Bedsores and their prevention is a large hospital expense. Two and one-half million patients are treated annually for pressure ulcers at a cost of between $9 billion and $11 billion. Divide three hundred million into nine billion, and that is about twenty-seven dollars per person.

Lawsuit judgments for bedsores developed in long-term-care facilities average $3.5 million; the largest judgment was $312 million. Not only do they take your money, but criminal charges may be filed if neglect is proven.

Factors leading to determination of neglect include the following:

- inadequate prevention
- poor documentation
- inadequate nutrition
- inadequate medical care
- no family notification
- poor care planning
- wound severity and outcome

There is an unavoidable ulcer category defined by the government's doublespeak as follows: an ulcer that occurs even though "the facility had evaluated the individual clinical condition and pressure ulcer risk factors; defined and implemented interventions that are consistent with individual needs, goals, and recognized standards of practice; monitored and evaluated the impact of the interventions; and revised the approaches as appropriate." In other words, it is an ulcer that occurs even if the hospital did everything appropriate to prevent the bedsore and kept meticulous records for the government to read—the latter being the most important.

Most long-term-care hospitals have the wound-care nurses take pictures of the wounds every Monday. Most of the wounds are diabetic foot ulcers.

If this much money is spent trying to prove that bedsores were taken care of properly, think how much money (your money) is spent on myriad other maladies.

Years ago, a senator suggested that a law be passed stating that the US Department of Agriculture could not have more employees than there were farmers. Today, perhaps, we need a law stating that a hospital cannot have more administrative personnel than there are patients.

Years ago, a hospital had an administrator and a head nurse; today there is a CEO (or president), a COO (chief operating officer), a CFO (chief financial officer), a nursing supervisor, an infection control nurse, a respiratory therapy supervisor, case managers, dieticians, and so on.

The chart had a face sheet, an order sheet, a graphic sheet, nurse's notes, doctor's notes, lab and x-ray reports, and an ECG, if done.

Today, the following items are common in patient charts:

- face sheet: This is a sheet bearing the patient's name, address, next of kin, and, above all, insurance information.
- orders: These are things doctors, now referred to as "caregivers," want done. We have nurse practitioners (nurse doctors). The system wants

more nurse practitioners because they erroneously think that money is being saved through their use. A surgeon complained that when nurse–doctors were staffing the emergency room on the weekend, many useless trips were made to evaluate patients with abdominal pain.

- progress notes made by the doctor: These are included so others reading the chart will know what is going on. Frequently, the doctor's writing is illegible, rendering the notes worthless, but that way the lawyers will not know whom to sue.
- patient education
- history, physical, and consults
- directives, consents, and admission data: These advanced directives by patients or guardians state whether the patient wants heroic measures to be taken if death is imminent.
- interdisciplinary care plan: This is doublespeak for more work by hospital employees, probably dictated by the government.
- procedure, anesthesia: This includes records of any operation that a patient might have had.
- reports of laboratory tests
- microbiology: Previously called bacteriology, this includes results of cultures, blood tests, urine tests, etc.
- blood administration: This is a record of blood transfusions.
- electrocardiogram (ECG), if done: In some long-term-care hospitals, only a strip rather than a

twelve-lead ECG is routinely put on the chart. The hospital may have to get the ECG read and won't get reimbursed for it. The hospital may get reimbursed if the nurse looks at the strip.

- radiology: This includes x-ray reports.
- pathology report
- graphics: This can include items relating to temperature, pulse, respiration, intake, and output.
- diabetic flowsheet: This is a record of blood sugar levels and insulin given.
- wounds: Pictures of wounds are kept to show progress.
- occupational therapy: This includes records related to the strengthening of the patient to do what is required for daily living.
- physical therapy: This includes records related to the strengthening of the patient.
- respiratory therapy: This includes records of oxygen and drugs blown into a patient's lungs and a record of ventilator settings if a patient is on a ventilator.
- nutrition: This includes an evaluation by a dietician.
- nursing: This includes nurses' notes evaluating a patient.
- case management: This relates to a nurse trying to expedite care (e.g., making sure that consultant sees the patient in a timely manner, rather than three days later). Hospitals are paid according to diagnosis-related code (DRC), which means that

the insurance company or the government will pay the hospital according to the diagnosis (e.g., pneumonia). A case manager makes sure that a patient doesn't dwell in the hospital because of uncoordinated care.

- referring facility records: These are records from another facility that are kept in the case of a patient being transferred to a hospital.

Today there is much more in a hospital chart than there used to be; therefore charts cost more money.

Hospitals are periodically inspected by the government (Medicare) or by a quasigovernmental organization, JACO. Much of what the inspectors demand be done is not that important for patient care, but it is expensive. For example, an inspector said that the handheld glucometer should be wiped off with alcohol between patients. A small strip of blotter paper with the patient's blood on it is put into the machine. When it was pointed out to the inspector that the machine does not touch the patient, the inspector said that the drop of blood might splatter. Splatter off a blotter? Really?

Computers are now replacing charts. Now the illegible doctor's writing can be read. It takes longer to put something in a computer, but the hospital chart can be retrieved from the doctor's office, also from the insurance company office, and from "Big Brother's" office.

After a patient is discharged from an acute-care hospital, he may be admitted to a long-term acute-care hospital to continue the care, which may involve long-term

IV antibiotics, physical therapy, dialysis, care of wounds, and so on. Most likely, such a patient will have "used up" his Medicare days at the regular hospital.

From the small slice of the country that the author has seen, most of the long-term acute-care hospital patients will have from three to six foreign medical graduate doctors seeing the patient every day. Many of the patients are receiving IV pain medicine every four to six hours because the government's "Pain Bill of Rights" states that everyone should be free of pain at all time. If you are not a junkie when you get here, you will be one before you leave. Many of the patients are vegetating on ventilators and would be better served in a hospice. If the patient—or more likely the patient's family—has not signed the government's advanced directives stating that the patient should be allowed to die in peace, then cardiac resuscitation or, more likely, resurrection will be attempted. This is expensive but uniformly futile.

The red cart will be rolled in. External chest compressions will be started. The ECG will show no heartbeat, a slow heartbeat, a regular heartbeat but no pulse (pulseless electrical activity [PEA]), or ventricular fibrillation (the heart muscle not contracting normally but more or less quivering).

If the patient is suffering from one of the above, ventricular fibrillation would be the best case, because the heart can be stopped with an electric shock and it will restart with a regular rhythm. If the patient is not rapidly resuscitated, an endotracheal tube will be placed for mechanical breathing. Epinephrine is given for the other problems. Atropine is given to speed up the heart by blocking the vagus nerve. If the node between the atrium (upper part of the heart) and the ventricle (lower part of the heart), the A-V node, is intact, atropine might work; otherwise atropine does not directly affect the heart.

After thirty minutes of cardiac resuscitation attempts (i.e., chest compression, epinephrine, vasopressin, and electric shock [if fibrillation is present]), efforts are stopped. A demented ninety- or ninety-nine-year-old patient will get the expensive and futile resuscitative attempt if the DNR (do not resuscitate) has not been signed or stated.

A security guard, until talked out of it, wanted an attempt to be made to resuscitate his mother because "God performs miracles." His mother was comatose from a brain metastasis from lung cancer. We have patients' families making medical decisions—wasteful medical decisions. The hospital doesn't mind. They make money—your, the taxpayer's, money.

It is very expensive for the taxpayer if no one is allowed to die in peace, without a resuscitative effort and an endotracheal tube. This is almost what we have in long-term acute-care hospitals.

If the patients in long-term acute-care hospitals don't get all the pain medicine that they want, the family might call Medicare or Medicaid and say, "They just let my mama lie there and suffer." Then the inspectors will come and disrupt the hospital for one or two days with their inspection. So hospital gives mama the pain shot that she doesn't need; it's easier.

The long-term acute-care hospitals and their doctors

cost the health-care system more money keeping patients "vegetating on ventilators" and trying to resuscitate them when they die. As it stands now, a patient may vegetate on a ventilator for the last two weeks of life, being seen daily by three to ten doctors, all of whom send a bill.

What can be done? When someone tries to address the problem, he is accused of wanting "death panels." Some doctors want to do this to make money. We need fewer money-grubbing doctors and more honest, better doctors.

The late William Larimer (Larry) Mellon entered Tulane Medical School at age forty. After graduating, Larry bought the Standard Fruit banana plantation, seventy to eighty miles from Port-au-Prince, Haiti; he built a hospital, which he and his wife, Gwen, with the aid of imported doctors, ran. Initially it cost Larry about $600,000 a year to run the hospital. Larry named the hospital Hospital Albert Schweitzer after Dr. Schweitzer, who ran a hospital in Africa, where babies were put on banana leaves for beds. Larry had visited Dr. Schweitzer.

At Hospital Albert Schweitzer in Deschapelles, Haiti, there were no stacks of papers to fill out and sign. The language, a patois called Creole, which the patients spoke, was unwritten. There were no lawyers, no insurance, no state boards, no worker's compensation, no joint commission, and no Medicare—just dedicated people doing their best to take care of the Haitian people was what was happening at Hospital Albert Schweitzer. This was infinitely cheaper than what was happening in the United States.

In the nursery at Hospital Albert Schweitzer, there were usually twenty to thirty newborn babies with neonatal tetanus. Most, if not all, of these babies died.

Larry thought that he could better help the people by teaching them public health—how to raise animals and such. The babies had tetanus because the mother or, more likely, the *bokar* (witch doctor) put mud on the umbilical cord at birth. When a patient was given worm pills, he might swallow them with river water.

Recently, the internet showed that Hospital Albert Schweitzer was operating with five hundred employees, a tribute to Larry and Gwen Mellon, two people who made a difference.

Farther away from Port-au-Prince, toward Cap-Haïtien, the tip of Haiti, where a fort was built waiting for the French to return, the late Caroline Bradshaw ran House of Hope, La Pointe Palmistes, where she cared for children with tuberculosis, especially tuberculosis of the spine. Every four months, she would load her van with several children with tuberculosis of the spine, Pott's disease, and take them to Hospital Albert Schweitzer, where one of a four-man Atlanta orthopedic group would do spinal fusions on those unfortunate children to keep their spines from collapsing more, paralyzing them.

According to Caroline Bradshaw's website, House of Hope, La Pointe des Palmistes, charged patients who came there, some as little as one penny. However, no one was turned away because of their inability to pay. The thought behind this was that if one paid, he would appreciate his care.

In one of the poorest nations, one pays; here in one of the richest nations, it is free. Maybe there should be a Medicaid co-pay.

Hospital Albert Schweitzer and House of Hope des Palmistes are extreme examples, but look at how much money could be saved if many of our laws and regulations were eliminated.

Hospitals have enormous expenses: medical liability insurance (usually the hospital gets sued when the doctor gets sued), worker's compensation insurance, infection control nurses to help prevent lawsuits, case managers to expedite patient care, accountants, food service, guards, medical records librarians, and so on. These added expenses are passed on to you, the consumer.

In one small hospital, premiums for the first million dollars of insurance were $900,000. The hospital self-insured the first million dollars. In other words there was no insurance.

When an anesthesiologist looked at the bill for his wife's delivery at a large hospital affiliated with a Christian church, he noticed that his wife had been charged for an epidural anesthetic as well as for a pudendal nerve block and charged for enough Phenergan (sedative) injections to sedate her until Whitsuntide. When the anesthesiologist asked the business office about the bill, he was told, "That is how we make money." This is the church stealing from you.

Hospitals can pad their bills because few people ever ask for an itemized bill, thinking erroneously that someone else is paying it.

A male x-ray technician at a small hospital came to a surgeon, a colleague of the x-ray technician, asking him how much he would charge to remove a lipoma (fat tumor) from his back. The x-ray technician said that an Indian surgeon wanted $900. For this much money, the lipoma would have to be removed in the hospital operating room rather than in the surgeon's office; an anesthesiologist might have sedated the patient, resulting in another bill, and the pathologist would have sent him a bill to tell him that this was a lipoma. The total bill would have been $2,000 to $4,000.

Small office procedures are done in the hospital as outpatient surgery or are done in a surgical center, because insurance companies pay very little for office procedures. The insurance cartel wants larger bills in order for them to charge larger premiums.

The second surgeon removed the x-ray technician's lipoma in the office and threw the lipoma in the garbage. There was no bill for the x-ray technician. This cost the surgeon ten to fifteen minutes of his time and a few dollars' worth of supplies, not counting the surgeon's rent, employee wages, phone call cost, and malpractice insurance.

This is but one example of the waste of medical resources. If every lump and bump is removed in a hospital, more money is wasted. The reply of the people removing lumps and bumps in a hospital is "There is no such thing as minor surgery, just minor surgeons."

These are extreme examples, but health-care costs could be greatly reduced without decreasing the quality of health care.

What kind of hospitals do we have?

Doctor-owned hospitals are usually built to make money, which lends itself to overutilization; occasionally a hospital is built to avoid the abuse of the doctors at the hospitals in which they practiced.

Investor-owned hospitals, which are occasionally privately owned and usually traded on the stock exchange, are another matter. The goal of a hospital company is to make money, as with other companies. If a company does not make money, it goes out of business. Some of these hospitals treat their staff doctors as rock stars to encourage them to help the hospital make money.

There are church-owned or church-named hospitals: Catholic, Methodist, Episcopal, and so on. The Baptist hospitals had to change their names in order to accept government money. The Hermann Hospital in Houston, donated by Mr. Hermann to take care of the indigent, became associated with the University of Texas Medical School and combined with the Baptist hospitals.

University hospitals are hospitals affiliated with and staffed by medical school staff and trainees.

Eleemosynary (charity) hospitals are run by a county or state and are staffed by interns and residents supervised by professors, providing excellent care for the indigent or those unfortunate to have been shot, stabbed, or in a wreck.

No matter the hospital, it is plagued with government regulations and defensive measures to prevent lawyers and their lawsuits.

Telemedicine

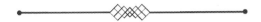

Telemedicine is sending a picture of yourself to your doctor or to a doctor. Some states want the teledoctor to have seen the patient, but they are getting around this. How long before your teleinformation goes to a computer instead of to a doctor?

We already had telemedicine in the past; the hospital nurse would call the patient's doctor and tell the doctor that the condition of the patient has changed. With modern telemedicine, the nurse sends a picture and the results of studies to an unknown doctor who hasn't seen the patient, resulting in another bill to the government or to an insurance company. Some patients may want their doctor to come check on them if their condition changes for the worse.

Some long-term acute-care hospitals are doing away with in-house doctors and replacing them with telemedicine. One purpose of in-house doctors is to keep the staff doctors from being called for little things: a patient falling out of bed, wanting a sleeping pill, needing orderly restraint, and so on. The telemedicine doctor could handle these small problems at a greater expense.

If the patient's telemedicine doctor is the patient's doctor, the staff doctor will have to answer his or her calls with more rapidity than has been done in the past.

Telemedicine may not always be the best for severely ill patients, but most are old and are unemployed, making them of little value to lawyers because Texas law limits the award for pain and suffering to $200,000. Wrongful death may be different!

Telemedicine may be good for remote patients or a dermatology revisit, but for hospitals, it may be just another source of income for hospitals.

Will the teledoctor change the treatment of the staff doctors without talking to him? Will the staff doctor change the treatment back when he sees the patient the next morning?

Government

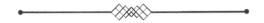

That which the government does is usually counterproductive.

The EMTALA law (Emergency Medical Treatment and Active Labor Act), dubbed the "anti-dumping law" by the phrasemongers and propagandists of the government-controlled media, states that a person can go to any hospital emergency room at any time and must be examined and stabilized without asking the patient about his or her ability to pay. The patient may not be transferred to another hospital without the receiving hospital (e.g., a charity hospital) and doctor agreeing to accept the patient.

A violation of the EMTALA law can result in a fine of $50,000 for doctors as well as for hospitals, and possibly a revocation of the ability to treat Medicare and Medicaid patients—in other words, it could possibly put hospitals out of business.

One of the first violations was a doctor sending a patient in labor from Victoria, Texas, to the state charity hospital in Galveston. Texas is a big place, and the patient delivered her baby before she reached Galveston. Victoria is about ninety miles from Houston, and Galveston another forty. Maybe $50,000 was cheaper than a $50 million dollar judgment for delivering a damaged baby—damaged because the mother had no prenatal care.

When a small hospital wants to transfer a nonresource patient to a charity city or county hospital where the patient belongs, the charity hospital asks that the patient's face sheet be faxed. The patient's face sheet shows that the patient has no insurance, skirting the EMATALA law. The charity hospital does not want your patient, because 30 percent of its budget is taken up with illegal aliens.

The pundits say that the immigration reform bill will overwhelm the health-care system. Now these people are taken care of through emergency rooms, which are much more expensive than being taken care of in a doctor's office. This is brought about by the EMTALA law.

Malpractice lawsuits prevent retired doctors from manning free clinics that could care for some of the indigent.

The following are some examples of EMTALA law abuses:

An ER doctor forgot to put his narcotics number on a prescription that he had given a patient who had come to the emergency room by ambulance. The patient called another ambulance to return her to the emergency room for the doctor to put his narcotics number on the prescription. The hospital probably charged for another ER visit. The pharmacist could have called the ER doctor. The ambulance charge is between $800 and $1,200. The emergency crews on the ambulances are instructed to pick up everyone who calls. It is probably much cheaper to pick up everyone who calls than to defend lawsuits.

A three-year-old girl dropped a can of tomato juice on her toe. An ambulance brought her to the emergency room. Her toe was not broken. She returned home in the car that could have brought her to the ER in the first place.

A lawyer who had been drinking was stopped by the highway patrol. The lawyer saw a disaster in the making; he complained of chest pain, faking a heart attack. When the ambulance came and wanted to take him to a nearby hospital with a cath lab and cardiologist, he made the ambulance take him to a very small hospital. After the ambulance had departed, when the ER personnel wanted to draw his blood and do an ECG, the lawyer got off the ER table and went out into the parking lot and left with a woman who was waiting for him. This was a slick way of beating a drunk-driving rap. The lawyer may have been an assistant district attorney.

An ambulance brought a large fifteen-year-old girl to the emergency room because she had been hit in the eye at school. There was no swelling—only a small streak on the lower lid. The patient was taken home in the car that could have brought her to the hospital in the first place.

A mother brought two young daughters to the ER because a bee had stung them. Mom had read that people die from insect bites. The two young girls were in no distress. They were running around playing in the waiting room. The nurse and the doctor told her that her daughters did not need to be seen in the ER. Mom called her husband, who said to have the young girls seen in the emergency room. The girls were written up; two bills were sent to Medicaid.

A dude came to the ER at 1:00 a.m. because of gonorrhea that he had had for two weeks. His last exposure had been a few hours prior; here was another ER customer. When the ambulance arrived at a downtown hospital, the patient got out of the ambulance, thanked the ambulance crew for the ride, and departed.

A Medicaid mom brought her child to the hospital emergency room on Friday, saying that she was sorry to have to come to the ER but her child had a fever and her doctor couldn't see her child until Tuesday. At twelve dollars a visit in California and eighteen dollars a visit in Texas for Medicaid patients, doctors have to limit the number of Medicaid patients that can be seen in one day; otherwise, the doctor will go broke.

A patient with a subdural hematoma, a blood clot around the brain, came to the emergency room of a very small hospital about sixty miles from Houston. A subdural hematoma can result from minor trauma weeks or months before symptoms occur. The few drops of blood around the brain and beneath the dura, an inelastic covering of the brain, break down and draw fluid into the area, causing the clot to expand, making the enlarging hematoma resemble a growing brain tumor. When the emergency room tried to transfer the patient to a hospital with a neurosurgeon, the hospital wanted a face sheet faxed that would show that the patient had no insurance, violating the EMTALA law, which states that the patient cannot be asked about his ability to pay. The emergency room doctor called nine hospitals before a hospital ninety miles from Houston agreed to take the patient. Were these other eight hospitals so full that they could not take this patient, who needed an emergency operation for a subdural hematoma?

Years ago in New Orleans, when a person, jailed for being drunk, did not sober up by the next morning, he was taken to a charity hospital. One such patient had a subdural hematoma. After surgery, the last thing that he remembered was that he was in Boston.

The operation for a subdural hematoma is usually simple—drill a hole in the skull and let the blood out. Sometimes the hematoma has existed so long that a sac has developed that needs to be removed.

Neurosurgeons do not want such a patient because not only will they not be paid, but they will also be sued if the patient already has brain damage. Patients with brain damage may need domiciliary care for thirty to forty years, requiring many millions of dollars; therefore, the plaintiff lawyer will sue everyone who remotely had anything to do with the patient, even though the doctor had nothing to do with causing the patient's problem. A neurosurgeon in Lufkin, Texas, is less likely to be sued than a neurosurgeon in Houston, Harris County, Texas, the epicenter of flawed justice.

The ill-conceived EMTALA law has turned emergency rooms into twenty-four-hour outpatient clinics and has turned ambulances into taxis, at great expense to the health-care system.

The hospitals don't mind seeing Medicaid and non-resource patients, because if the hospital sees enough of these patients, the hospital comes under the government's disproportionate share program and receives money from the government.

The EMTALA law and the Disproportionate Share Program give us universal coverage and universal payment—that is, government medical care.

Patient's Pain Bill of Rights

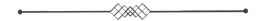

The federal government has given us the Patient's Pain Bill of Rights, which decrees that patients should be free of pain.

Nurses are required to visit the patients periodically and show them a cartoon with faces ranging from a smile to a frown. The patient is required to pick out the face that best describes his or her pain. The patient may not need pain medication, but to accommodate the nurse, he or she may pick out a face showing some pain.

If one has a big operation or is run over by a truck, one should have some pain. Pain doctors differ. They think that if one's pain is not controlled at all times, one might have chronic pain. If a patient is sedated at all times, he or she doesn't breathe deeply, which causes pneumonia and atelectasis (unexpanded lung); the patient doesn't move his or her legs and gets clots in the veins—clots that may break off and go into the lungs and kill the patient—and the patient experiences decreased intestinal peristalsis, which causes him or her to remain in the hospital longer if he or she had an abdominal operation.

Patients know that when they enter a long-term

acute-care hospital, they can get all the narcotics that they want. Many patients get IV narcotics twenty-four hours a day.

Now we have a new specialist, the pain specialist, who may manage the pain of hospitalized patients, inject patients in a hospital setting, or see patients in his or her office.

The hospital visits are to manage the patient's pain. Outpatient injections are usually a local anesthetic mixed with cortisone to reduce inflammation. Many of the outpatient pain doctors flood the streets with narcotics (as in the case of pill mills).

The hospital pain specialist is just another doctor to come by, see the patient, and send a bill. If a surgeon has operated on ten to twenty thousand patients, he or she should be able to manage the patient's pain. Pain specialists say that 50 percent of surgery patients receive an inadequate amount of narcotics. The pain specialists allege that not only do the patients suffer unnecessary pain but also that the pain may remain as chronic pain after the patient leaves the hospital. If all you have is a hammer, everything looks like a nail.

Statistics don't lie; statisticians do. A recent newspaper article said that the government was going to base Medicare reimbursements on the hospitals' results in treating patients. One measurement would be how many patients died shortly after leaving the hospital. This would prevent hospitals from skewing their mortality figures by sending patients to a hospice to die.

The article also said that how soon after an operation

a patient received antibiotics would be considered. Prophylactic antibiotics should be given before surgery, not after surgery. This statement makes one wonder if these clowns have any idea what they are speaking about.

To measure a hospital's results in treating patients, one would have to take into account what kind of patients are being treated. One hospital may be in a more affluent part of town where patients are healthier and take better care of themselves. Another hospital may be in an area where patients are overweight, don't control their diabetes, and can't afford their medicines.

What are the measurements of the results? Are we comparing a twenty-year-old with a ninety-year-old, both of whom had strangulated hernias? Are we comparing a forty-year-old man who had his first heart attack with a seventy-year-old man who had his third heart attack?

The hospital wrote a doctor telling him that he had two subcutaneous wound infections in one month. One elderly patient had had a ruptured cecal cancer at the base of his appendix for twenty-four hours before he came to the hospital. The other patient had a ruptured colon and required cortisone because two weeks prior, he had been in the hospital on a ventilator and taking cortisone.

If any financial benefit were to be derived from this program, it would not pay for the bureaucrats running it.

This program comes under one of Professor C. Northcoat Parkinson's laws—"Bureaucrats make work for each other."

HIPAA

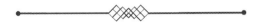

The Health Information Portability and Accountability Act has to do with transferring one's health insurance. It also has to do with privacy.

If an emergency room doctor in a small hospital sends an unusual and perplexing case to a large hospital, the doctor can't find out the outcome of the case. One can't call and see if one's friend is still in the hospital or if the friend was ever there in the first place.

Independent Physicians Association

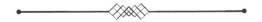

The Independent Physicians Association (IPA) is an organization owned by doctors. The plan was to give the doctors a fixed amount of money to take care of a fixed number of patients (i.e., capitation). The patients were signed up by primary care doctors, who signed up specialists. The government plan was to pay the doctors to keep the patients well. Well, some of the doctors kept the money and murdered the patients with neglect.

One plan signed up Medicare patients and paid for their medicine. With a little thought, these Medicare victims should have been able to figure out that if a group of doctors took a slice out of the original Medicare money, that there would be less for the patients.

Today the same applies to insurance companies that want to sell you their Medicare plan that gives you medicine and other benefits not furnished by traditional Medicare. You are not told that you have to use their doctor and their hospital, not the first-class hospital downtown.

A man in his late forties vomited blood for six months before his IPA primary doctor had a (paid) gastroenterologist gastroscope the patient and diagnose his stomach cancer. Stomach cancer does not have a good survival rate. A six-month delay decreases the patient's chance of survival.

A primary care doctor did not do routine PAP smears and mammograms on the female patients in her panel.

A patient in her seventies was bleeding from a large stomach cancer. The IPA did not want her to have surgery, but the surgeon, also capitated, operated on her anyway, giving the patient several months of life rather than letting her bleed herself into the grave. Elderly patients don't do well with total gastrectomies. Maybe the IPA was right, but some of us are not God.

Advanced Directives

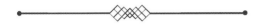

When one enters a hospital, one is required to fill out advanced directives stating whether or not one wants heroic measures instituted if death is imminent. The patient may give power of attorney to a family member to make this decision.

This results in expensive attempts at cardiac resuscitation, more likely resurrection, on demented ninety-nine-year-old patients. If possible, the patient will be intubated during the resurrection attempt. This adds another expense to the already considerable expense of the resuscitative effort. Today it appears that no one can die without someone pounding on his or her chest and someone sticking an endotracheal tube in him or her.

After an endotracheal tube is put into a patient, an x-ray is taken to check the tube placement. If the tube is put in too far, it will go into the right lung, leaving the left lung getting no air. Tube placement can be checked at the time of placement by listening to air coming into both lungs. Air coming into both lungs and the tube going in less than 23 centimeters in an average-size patient can assure one of correct tube placement.

If no one can die without cardiac resuscitation and an endotracheal tube and an unnecessary x-ray, this is costing the health-care system much money. The only beneficiaries are the hospitals, the doctors, and the Mercedes and Porsche dealerships. As usual, the taxpayers are the losers.

The hospitals say that they will be sued if resuscitative efforts aren't made on patients without "DNR" ("do not resuscitate") on their chart.

On nurses' testimony, two doctors in California were charged with murder for turning off a patient's ventilator. Justice is a big business—a business unimpeded by the law. The doctors had to hire expensive lawyers to defend themselves.

A patient signed a DNR order to ensure no heroic efforts would be made if death was imminent, but one of her several daughters wanted to keep her on the ventilator, where the patient had been for the past few weeks. The Social Security checks were still coming.

After an abdominal aneurysm surgery, while in the recovery room, an internist put the patient on a PCA pump for narcotics. When the patient's respiratory rate slowed to eight breaths per minute, the foreign graduate nurse was going to let the patient die because he signed a DNR. One of the surgeons came by and reversed the narcotics with Narcan.

Here is a hypothetical case: An eighty-plus-year-old patient was admitted to the hospital because of a compression fracture of his spine. He called his friend and said, "Come get me out of here; they are going to kill me. I want to leave everything to you." Before the friend could get him out of the hospital, the patient died. He had been put on a ventilator which was turned off because he had signed the DNR advanced directives. This occurred in 2010, when there was no inheritance tax. Two weeks later, the inheritance tax was 30 percent. The patient's timely demise saved his heirs $27 million. His estate was worth $90 million.

A man with kidney cancer, diabetes, renal failure, and respiratory failure had low blood pressure and was on two vasopressors (medicine to keep blood pressure up), a ventilator, and dialysis. He was comatose and appeared dead. He received a resuscitative effort because his wife wanted it. He was essentially a heart-and-lung preparation. Ten doctors were seeing him.

This scenario is played out many times daily in the United States, costing the health-care system (i.e., taxpayers) much money.

When you enter a hospital, do not sign an advanced directive; a nurse who graduated from some unknown foreign land may needlessly let you die, or your family might polish you off for your estate; anyway, if you are dead, it doesn't matter if people are pounding on your chest, putting drugs in your veins, or putting a tube in your throat. Besides, you won't have to worry about those clowns wrecking the health-care system.

JACO

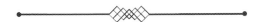

Formerly JCAH (Joint Commission on Accreditation of Hospitals) might be a quasigovernmental organization because Medicare inspectors follow in their footsteps. Hospitals have to be accredited in order to do business with Medicare and insurance companies.

Much of what the inspectors want done does not directly involve patient care; nevertheless, it adds to the patient's hospital bill. Now inspectors are inspecting doctor's offices, resulting in more expenses.

Texas State Board of Medical Examiners

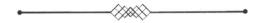

The Texas State Board of Medical Examiners, lapdogs of the trial lawyers, have swallowed the line "The medical malpractice crisis is caused by a few bad doctors, and all that needs to be done is to get rid of these bad apples," put out by the government propaganda ministry (ABC, CBS, NBC, CNN, etc.), which makes Dr. Goebbels look like a Boy Scout.

The phrasemongers and propagandists don't mention that some of the world's best doctors have many lawsuits.

In their quest to stamp out "bad doctors," the state board has disregarded the Constitution.

All doctors and all lawyers are required to post a sign written in English and Spanish in their offices giving the number of the state board to call if they have a complaint against the doctor. This maneuver increases lawsuits by suggesting that the doctor does things that require a complaint.

Requiring that a doctor post a sign advertising for

business probably violates the Thirteenth Amendment against involuntary servitude.

The doctor's offices have large state board signs. The lawyer's office is usually dimly lit and expensively decorated, with the state board sign in a small picture frame sitting on a table, obscured by an expensive lamp.

When a patient complains to the state licensure board, either because the patient is dissatisfied, because the patient's lawyer told him to do so, or because one of the doctor's competitors or detractors told him to do so, the state board writes the doctor, who is now referred to as a licensee, to reply to the complaint in writing, violating the doctor's (licensee) Fifth Amendment right against self-incrimination.

The state board notifies the hospitals in the state that they are investigating the doctor, no matter how frivolous the complaint. The hospital then writes the doctor, asking him why he is being investigated by the Texas State Board of Medical Examiners. Some doctors send the hospital a copy of the Fifth Amendment and tell the hospital that they do not want to answer their question. This takes care of the hospital.

The state board will not tell the doctor who filed the complaint against him, violating *Pointer v. State of Texas*, which ruled that a person has a right to cross-examine the accuser. The board's answer is that this is only an investigation, but the insurance company may increase the doctor's rates. The board alleges that they are the accuser.

If the board is the accuser, then there must have been an informant. If it has not been repealed, *Firi v. United*

States (1965) held that a person can know the identity of the informant if it is necessary for his or her defense.

The board further states that if there is a hearing, then the licensee will be granted due process, which is broadly defined as fairness. One is entitled to due process at all times!

The board then says that if there is a hearing, then the licensee (doctor) can cross-examine the complainant *if the complainant decides to appear.*

All this investigation takes longer than OJ's first trial, and when the board tells him what he already knew—that the complaint was without merit—they throw in that this would be a good time for the doctor to evaluate the way that he practices medicine, inferring that it is the doctor's fault that some nut, a lawyer, or one of his competitors got the lapdogs to waste so much of the taxpayer's money investigating him.

A doctor, walking through the hospital, was spoken to by an old patient. The doctor could not remember her, but he passed pleasantries. Several days later, the doctor received a letter from the State Board of Medical Examiners accusing him of practicing medicine against the welfare of the people of the State of Texas by abandoning a patient.

As it turned out, ten years prior the doctor had removed a colon cancer and placed a venous access port for chemotherapy for the patient with whom he had passed pleasantries in the hospital corridor. This was the complainant.

About six months after the operation, her oncologist did a chest x-ray that showed a piece of wire in the patient's heart. When placing a venous access port, the introducer is threaded over a wire.

A cardiologist removed the wire without incident, but the patient remained in the hospital overnight for observation. Several months later, the doctor who had placed the port learned of the incident.

When a venous access catheter is placed, an x-ray is taken to check its position. No wire was seen at that time. Most likely someone had tried to unstop the catheter by passing a wire through a needle that had been inserted into the port chamber and the needle cut the wire when the wire was pulled out. Ports have been replaced by PICC lines—IVs placed in the upper arm using an ultrasound. The catheter is threaded into the vena cava.

The patient had answered a lawyer's newspaper ad. When she called the lawyer, she was told to report the doctor to the Texas State Board of Medical Examiners. This she did, complaining that her surgeon had abandoned her ten years ago when she spent the night in the hospital and he did not come visit her. The surgeon's not knowing that she was hospitalized was of no consequence.

This occurred at the time when three thousand medical malpractice suits for nine thousand doctors were filed in Harris County, Texas, in the four to six weeks before a constitutional amendment limiting damages for pain and suffering came into effect.

Complaints to the Texas State Board of Medical Examiners should be added to the list of things for which there is no statute of limitation: murder, military desertion, plagiarism by a college student, and so on.

This is another assault on doctors to achieve government (insurance company) medicine.

A fifteen-year-old girl fell out of the back of a pickup truck. She had a scalp laceration that was sutured by the emergency room doctor. A CT scan of the head was done even though she was never unconscious. She was admitted overnight for observation. The next day, the admitting doctor wanted to discharge the patient, but the Medicaid mom wanted her daughter to remain hospitalized. The next day, the doctor wanted to discharge the patient, but the patient's mother again insisted that her daughter remain hospitalized. Mom had a very expensive babysitter. The following day, the mother again wanted her daughter to remain hospitalized, but this time the doctor insisted that the patient be discharged. The irate mom wrote the hospital, calling the doctor a bigot, among other things.

Two days after discharge, the patient was seen in the doctor's office. The doctor got this patient because he was covering for his colleague, who had to take emergency room patients as a condition for being on the hospital staff.

The wound was infected. The braided silk sutures were removed because they harbored bacteria. The mother was asked to put hot compresses on the wound and to return to the office in a few days. The wound dehisced (broke open), and the mother took the patient to another doctor, who did another CT scan of the child's head, probably using a machine in which he had a financial interest. He told the mother that the sutures should have been left in place for twelve days.

Three years later, the mother called the doctor's office asking for her daughter's medical records. The office records were sent, but the mother said that she could not read them. The doctor's employee said that this was all they had. The Texas Board of Medical Examiners wrote the doctor that three years prior he had practiced medicine against the welfare of the people by prematurely removing scalp sutures.

The doctor called the state board and asked how long infected braided silk sutures should be left in an infected scalp wound. Their answer was "We can't tell you, but you are accused of taking them out too soon. Monofilament sutures could have been left in place." The doctor did not suture the scalp wound; the emergency room doctor did. The doctor could have used monofilament sutures. Perhaps the ER had been out of monofilament sutures.

This assault on the doctors by the licensure board and by the insurance cartel and their lackey lawyers is part of the grand design of an insurance cartel to drive the doctors into government health care. All this is aided by their propaganda ministry.

Recently, with Governor Rick Perry at the helm, Texas passed an antiabortion bill stating that abortions cannot be done after twenty weeks of gestation and that the doctor performing the abortion must be on the staff of a hospital within thirty miles.

To be on a hospital staff, a doctor is required to have medical liability insurance (malpractice insurance), an amount dictated by the hospital. An ob-gyn specialist may pay $100,000 to $200,000 a year for malpractice insurance. Perhaps this is lower after the Texas Tort Reform Amendment.

As stated elsewhere, the insurance cartel is writing claims made rather than occurrence policies. An occurrence policy covers the time from the occurrences of alleged malpractice. Claims made policies cover from the time that the claim was made. The statute of limitations for malpractice is two years, plus another forty-five days for additional parties. One has to renew one's malpractice policy every year. Most malpractice suits are not filed until one year after the occurrence. The doctor is not really insured if his or her policy is not renewed.

Most hospitals require its staff doctors to be on emergency room call to treat and admit patients who have no doctor, insurance, or money. These patients are a liability nightmare: patients with no prenatal care who show up in labor at the emergency room, patients who delay seeking medical treatment because of lack of resources, patients who have pursued an unhealthy lifestyle, and so on.

A number of years ago, Texas bureaucrats, in their infinite wisdom, required hospitals to get a certificate of need before the hospital could buy a piece of equipment. To get this certificate, the hospital lawyer had to attend a meeting in Austin, the capital, and explain why the equipment was needed, while the hospital's competitors sent their lawyers to show why the equipment wasn't needed. When a hospital wanted to replace a worn-out $90,000 x-ray machine, the legal fees were over $90,000.

This silly regulation allowed investors to set up CT scans, paying doctors (investors) to send business.

When it was on the front page of the newspaper that a handsome young investor had taken a woman on the committee that grants certificates of need to Mexico for a weekend in order to get a certificate of need to build a hospital, the certificate of need program was scrapped.

Many years ago, the professor of obstetrics and gynecology had a large, perhaps the largest in the world, number of vena cava and ovarian vein ligations for septic pelvic thrombophlebitis, as a result of abortions done by midwives, probably on kitchen tables. These hapless women will forever have swollen legs. Today we have more and better antibiotics, and fewer midwives doing abortions.

Governor, we are up to our hips in the babies of unmarried teenage mothers!

The government, or its minions, has decreed that if a patient is to be restrained because the patient will pull out his or her lines or because the patient will fall out of bed, an order to restrain the patient must be written by the doctor and repeated along with a note daily thereafter. Nurses know which patients need restraint. More paperwork!

Insurance Lawyers

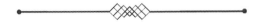

Medical liability insurance has done more to wreck our health care than any other thing.

With the help of the propaganda ministry, the insurance oligarchs were able to increase medical premiums to an astronomical level. This was done by unmeritorious lawsuits, which were milked for thousands of dollars before being dropped or settled for nuisance amounts. The next year, everyone's premiums were increased!

A case in point: A plastic surgeon did liposuction in a patient's neck, injuring the spinal accessory nerve, which was probably bruised. This nerve comes from the brain, at one point passing just beneath the skin of the neck. The nerve innervates the muscles that hold the scapula to the body; therefore, when the spinal accessory nerve is damaged, the result is a "winged scapula." The shoulder blade sticks out from the chest. Little trauma is required to cause the nerve not to function for several weeks or several months.

The patient sued the plastic surgeon for damaging her

nerve, and she sued the anesthesiologist for holding her neck in the wrong position.

The anesthesiologist was dropped from the suit without ever being deposed or going to court. The anesthesiologist's insurance carrier wrote him a letter telling him that they had spent $90,000 defending him. That $90,000, divided by $300 per hour, is 300. Three hundred hours divided by 24, the number of hours in a day, is 12.5. This means that to earn $90,000 working for $300 per hour, the lawyers would have to work 24 hours a day for 12.5 days.

Why would an insurance company pay a lawyer so much money for so little work? Could it be greed? Could it be that the insurance company wanted to increase every doctor's rates next year?

The anesthesiologist will forever have this lawsuit on his record—a record that will be used by insurance carriers when writing him insurance policies and by the hospital granting him hospital privileges. The propaganda ministry will label him one of those bad doctors that are causing the health-care crisis.

At trial, the plastic surgeon prevailed. No doubt the patient's spinal accessory nerve had regenerated by then.

If $90,000 was spent defending the anesthesiologist, who did nothing, how much was spent defending the plastic surgeon? Hundreds of thousands of dollars were sucked out of the health-care system.

In another case, when an unmeritorious malpractice lawsuit was filed against a doctor, a video deposition was taken before the suit was dropped. At the video deposition, there were six lawyers asking inane questions and taking many breaks. Six lawyers at $300 an hour is $1,800 an hour. A twenty-minute break costs the system $600.

One doctor's video deposition was put on the evening news, violating the Thirteenth Amendment against involuntary servitude. They were making the doctor, through his images, sell beer, dog food, and Stayfree maxi pads.

A doctor was insured by a company that capitated its lawyers. "Capitated" is the payment to lawyers of a certain amount per doctor to defend the doctors whether the doctors are sued or not.

When one of its doctors had an unmeritorious suit filed against him, a summary judgment was obtained in a New York minute.

Had the doctor not been insured by a company that capitated its lawyers, many thousands of dollars would have been wasted, as in the above cases.

The practices of fomenting and milking malpractice suits have allowed the insurance cartel to raise medical liability premiums to an unsustainable level. A Philadelphia neurosurgeon pays $350,000 a year in malpractice premiums; cardiac surgeons, $100,000; obstetricians, $100,000–$200,000. Patients can't afford it. All inflation ends when people can no longer afford it. Now we are there. So what do we do? Turn to the government, of course. Perhaps people can no longer afford our government.

The CEO of UnitedHealthcare was reported to have $1.7 billion in unexercised stock options. There were complaints. He settled for $5 million a year. UnitedHealthcare ran the Medicaid health maintenance organization (HMO) Evercare, dubbed "Nevercare" by the doctors. One had to get permission from a person in an office downtown to close a bed sore or do a skin graft. Frequently, permission was not forthcoming. Perhaps this is where the CEO's money came from.

A young lady finished law school and joined a law firm, where she was told to bill the client even if she was just thinking about the case. She quit and started selling wedding dresses over the internet, making more money.

To be on a hospital staff, a doctor is required to buy medical liability insurance in an amount designated by the hospital. If one operates on or treats sick people, one has to work in a hospital.

A doctor paid his enormous malpractice insurance premiums in installments. The insurance company went bankrupt, causing the doctor to buy insurance from another company. The original company had sold the doctor's note to another company; the insurance company sued the doctor to pay for the original policy, although he was not insured and had already bought another policy. Nice fellows, these insurance oligarchs.

There are two types of malpractice insurance policies: occurrence and claims made. An occurrence policy insures the doctor from the time the alleged malpractice occurred. The claims made policy insures the doctor from the time the claim was made. The statute of limitations for malpractice is two years, and another forty-five days for additional parties to the suit.

Most medical malpractice suits are not filed until one year after the occurrence. If one has a malpractice occurrence, the insurance company could choose not to renew the policy, leaving the doctor with the claims made policy uninsured. Insurance companies are now writing claims made policies. This amounts to doctors paying tribute to the insurance cartel for the ability to practice medicine. Nice fellows, these insurance oligarchs!

What does it mean for a doctor to be sued? First, if you are in Texas, a lanky dude wearing a cowperson hat with an Alpine Crush block in it, the kind worn by President Lyndon Johnson and Governor John Connally, hands you some legal papers stating the awful things that you did to this person, and he wants you to give him a zillion dollars.

The hapless doctor will have to call his malpractice insurance carrier, which will assign him a lawyer. The doctor must hope the lawyer will be from a firm that has given $30,000 to the judge's campaign. Thirty thousand is the maximum amount that a law firm can contribute to a judge's campaign in Harris County, Texas. Unwritten, it may be the minimum amount also.

The assigned lawyer will meet with the doctor, messing up the doctor's afternoon. A deposition may be taken, messing up the doctor's entire day.

If the case goes to trial, two weeks of the good doctor's time will be wasted. Lawyers derisively refer to doctors as "the good doctor." If there is a trial, which is unlikely, the good doctor will be completely out of his element. The lawyer frequently goes to trial; the good doctor, never.

The only salvation for the good doctor is that he knows infinitely more about medicine than does the lawyer. That is, unless the lawyer is really good and learned the medicine.

Whether this lawsuit is dropped without a deposition or goes to trial, it will be on the good doctor's record forever. Every time he reapplies for hospital staff or malpractice insurance, he will be asked to list malpractice suits against him. He might as well have it tattooed on his arm, as if he had been in a concentration camp.

A doctor's employee filled out the doctor's yearly reapplication for a hospital. To the question "Have you had any malpractice lawsuits?" she replied "no," meaning "since I filled this out last year." The hospital already knew of lawsuits that had been filed against him. When the doctor moved to California, a hospital to which he applied turned him down because the hospital mentioned above said that the doctor had falsified his staff application. It pays to know who is trying to foul you.

The patient gets about 17 percent of the malpractice insurance premiums. The rest goes to the insurance companies, the lawyers, and the expert witnesses. There are doting old fool doctors living in Sun City who advertise in the bar journals to be expert witnesses. They will say anything for $10,000. Texas passed a law requiring medical expert witnesses to have Texas medical licenses and be specialists in the fields in which they are testifying.

"The malpractice insurance crisis is caused by a few bad doctors, and all we need to do is get rid of these bad apples" is the refrain sung by the government's phrasemongers and propagandists, to wit: ABC, NBC, CBS, CNN, the *New York Times*, and so on.

The propagandists haven't explained why some of the best doctors in the world have so many malpractice suits filed against them. Nor have they explained why there were three thousand lawsuits filed against about nine thousand doctors in Harris County, Texas, four to six weeks before the Tort Reform Amendment came into effect. Tort reform was an amendment to the Texas constitution. The trial lawyers could have changed a law; repealing an amendment is more difficult.

Several years ago, Dr. Denton Cooley, the best heart surgeon in the world, had seventy civil suits—a few not for malpractice. A few years later, when a lawyer checked at the courthouse, the list of suits Dr. Cooley was involved in covered seven computer screens. The lawyer did not count them.

Dr. Cooley probably did ten times the number of operations as did the average heart surgeon. Also, Dr. Cooley was sued for implanting an artificial heart in a patient who died. No doubt the patient was near death. Dr. Cooley prevailed, but the case cost many thousands of dollars. The lawyers' names were in the paper daily.

The late Dr. Michael DeBakey, the premier surgeon in the country, had ten malpractice suits. Dr. DeBakey was summoned to Russia to preside over Premier Yeltsin's heart surgery. Apparently the Russian surgeons wanted insurance against being sent to Siberia if Premier Yeltsin's operation did not turn out well.

Dr. DeBakey had at least one more malpractice suit.

His dentist sued him. Dr. DeBakey, then in his nineties and retired from doing surgery, advised his dentist to have his abdominal aneurysm attended to. When an abdominal aortic aneurysm reaches 5 centimeters, it tends to increase in size, and in many cases, it ruptures. A ruptured abdominal aneurysm has a significant risk of mortality, even if one is parked in front of a large hospital when it happens.

The dentist alleged that he was impotent following the operation—a known complication of abdominal aneurysm surgery—and that Dr. DeBakey did not tell him of this.

Dr. DeBakey was under no duty to describe the operation and its complications. I am certain that this was explained to the dentist when he signed the surgical consent form.

Using a recorder, the explanation of the patient's heart operation to be done (informed consent) was recorded. Three months after the operation, the patients remembered 10 percent of the information given them.

Dr. DeBakey's trial took two weeks, with everyone's name in the newspaper every day. Why was this case not dismissed?

At trial, Dr. DeBakey prevailed when his lawyer extolled the virtues of Viagra.

Fifty years ago, a doctor had an office over a drugstore. He charged two dollars a visit, and he put the money in a cigar box. If someone was sick, he sent them to a hospital. There were no computers, no insurance, and no state inspectors telling him to post a sign in English and

Spanish giving patients the number of the state licensure board, where complaints against the doctor could be filed.

Today a young college graduate had a vaginal discharge and called a gynecologist's office that told her an office visit would cost $200. The young lady had not yet found a job and was no longer on her family's insurance. If the gynecologist delivered babies, his malpractice insurance could be $100,000 to $200,000. His office overhead could approach 50 percent. The young lady was cured with some over-the-counter Monistat.

An emergency room called a neurosurgeon and asked him to come see a quadriplegic patient. The neurosurgeon said that he did not see quadriplegic patients because they all sued. The emergency room called him back and said, "Please come see this quadriplegic patient; no one else will come." The neurosurgeon went to the emergency room and saw the quadriplegic patient. She sued him.

An intensive care nurse was dating a lawyer who kept asking her to "send him a quad." Damages were so severe that a lawyer could retire on a "quad case."

An ophthalmologist practicing in northern Mississippi wanted to slow down by no longer doing surgery but instead working in the office. He couldn't, as the malpractice premiums were too high. The ophthalmologist said that there was a county seat in northern Mississippi that had more lawsuits filed than there were people living in the county seat. Apparently a person would get a Fen-Phen prescription in California, get it filled in northern Mississippi, take a few pills, and then sue the pharmaceutical company because the drug caused him to have heart failure.

In one case, even though expert testimony said that the plaintiff did not have heart failure, the jury awarded the plaintiff $6 million because he was afraid that he might get heart failure.

A juror asked the plaintiff for a tip for being so generous with the insurance company's money—your money.

Is the country crazy to let the insurance oligarchs and their lackey lawyers do this?

In the Rio Grande Valley of Texas, there are numerous wrecks on the highway that parallels the Rio Grande. An emergency room doctor in one hospital said that he had two head injury patients die without having been seen by a neurosurgeon. There were so many malpractice suits in the Rio Grande Valley that neurosurgeons don't want to practice there.

At an outlying hospital in a Texas city, the only infectious disease group will not see patients under twenty-one years of age because the statute of limitation for children runs until the child is twenty-one years old or twenty-one years plus two years. The surgeons use this as an excuse not to operate on children who have appendicitis, because if the child developed an infection, the lawyers would ask, "Why didn't you call an infectious disease specialist?" Most appendectomies are done at night, and the pay is so scant that it is not worth staying up half the night, especially when one has to get up the next morning and operate on patients.

A pathologist read a frozen section slide as cancer. The surgeon removed the woman's breast. After her breast had been removed, she sent the slides to her brother, a pathologist in another city. The pathologist and his colleagues said that the slides showed no cancer. All the colleagues of the original pathologist agreed with him, saying that it was cancer.

The patient sued the original pathologist and received a $3 million judgment. The pathologist had $1 million in malpractice insurance. The surgeon was also sued. While looking at his bank statements, the original pathologist died of a heart attack.

The law (either statutory or case) says that if a pathologist makes a slide correctly and looks at the slide correctly, he is not negligent. Even though the pathologist in this case made an incorrect diagnosis, he was not guilty of malpractice.

The original specimen was lost, which might have inflamed the jury; however, what subsequent sections showed should be irrelevant.

Harris County, Texas, is the epicenter of flawed justice. As stated previously, law firms are limited to $30,000 when contributing to a judge's election campaign.

As a result of this case, some surgeons quit doing frozen sections, resulting in women with breast cancer having two anesthetics and two operations. Stereotactic needle biopsies now have solved this problem.

As a result of this case, breast biopsy slides were sent to the famous M. D. Anderson Cancer Hospital for reading. The pathologist at M. D. Anderson became overwhelmed and would no longer read the slides unless the patient came along.

The system murdered this pathologist, who in addition to being an excellent pathologist, was a very nice person.

A call came in to the hospital dining room, where doctors were eating lunch, for a surgeon to come repair an iliac artery that had been punctured with an old-style trocar while a gynecologist was doing laparoscopy. A newer trocar with a safety device might have prevented this mishap. The arteries, covered by the peritoneum and under pressure from the carbon dioxide used to distend the abdomen to do laparoscopy, don't spurt blood as they might in an arm or a leg.

When the surgeon went to repair the artery, another surgeon offered to assist him. The surgeon said, "Don't come. They are going to sue us all." The assistant went anyway. If an artery is severed completely, five hands are usually needed: two hands to hold the ends together, one to sew, one to pick up the thing that is being sewn, and one to follow holding the suture to keep the suture line from being loose.

The insurance carrier of the gynecologist, the anesthesiologist, and his nurse assistant paid damages to the plaintiff.

As predicted, the plaintiff lawyer, an ersatz Jew, wrote the required notification letter stating that he was going to sue the surgeon, a real Jew, and his assistant. The surgeon said that he called the plaintiff lawyer and told him that he, the surgeon, had in no way harmed his client and that he had been in the Israeli Army and that he had better not fool with him. Most likely, the surgeon said that he had been in the Mossad and he had better not fool with him. The Mossad is the secret Israeli organization that makes the CIA, MI-5 and 6, and the old KGB look like Boy Scouts. The plaintiff lawyer demurred.

The assistant surgeon wrote the plaintiff lawyer, telling him that he could not remember whether his insurance carrier was the one that was in receivership or the one that was bankrupt. No largess from the insurance oligarchs!

Had the plaintiff lawyer filed suits against the surgeon and his assistant, there would have been depositions, letters, and phone calls for several months before the cases were dropped or settled for a nuisance amount. The suits would forever be on the doctor's record, labeling him as one of the bad doctors wrecking the health-care system.

Florida was considering a law that would take a doctor's license if he had three malpractice judgments against him. If the law did not include settlements, then much money would be extorted from the doctors. Floridians must have a short memory. A few years ago, no neurosurgeon would go to an emergency room in Dade County (Miami) because of lawsuits. If this law were passed, doctors in litigious specialties (e.g., obstetrics and neurosurgery) would leave Florida or wouldn't go there in the first place.

In Florida, bedsores can be a criminal offense—abuse of an old person. Patients with low serum albumens get bedsores. Perhaps doctors and nursing homes won't accept old patients with low serum albumens.

There was an article lamenting the fact that an

emergency room doctor's name was not put in the medical malpractice data bank because the hospital paid the $70 million judgment for sending home from the emergency room a patient with a headache. The patient ruptured a berry aneurysm in her head and was severely damaged neurologically. This patient could have used a CT scan. Now everyone with a headache will get a CT scan.

Governor Perry of Texas wants to introduce a loser-pays law for lawsuits. A past president of the Harris County Medical Society said that this had been tried for malpractice suits in Florida and it did not work because when the defendant doctor lost, it was $200,000, and when the plaintiff lost it was $20,000.

There was a newspaper article lamenting the decrease in the number of mammograms being done. The reason mammograms are not being done is that mammograms are a generator of lawsuits and doctors don't want to do them.

The insurance cartel and their lackey lawyers haven't limited their thievery to the health-care system. A tank truck skidded off the road in the Rio Grande Valley in Texas and plowed into a group of people, killing and injuring several. A $10 million judgment was rendered against the company in west Texas that made the tank ten years previously. The company had a reputation for making superior tanks. The company's insurance cost went from $2,000 a year to $600,000 a year. The owner laid off three hundred employees, closed the plant, had a heart attack, and died. Where do these jurors think this money comes from?

The feds closed a small bank in an outlying town and sold it to a politically connected large bank in the city for $225,000, although the owners had been offered $7 million. The feds sued the bank board. The bank board never saw a US attorney, dealing only with private lawyers who were paid $3 million by the government. The case was settled with a nondisclosure clause.

If US attorneys can dole out $3 million of legal work to their friends or to their future law partners, might not the US attorneys look for people to prosecute whether they need prosecuting or not?

How much of the taxpayer's money, if any, was spent hiring private attorneys to persecute Martha Stewart, John Edwards, and Roger Clemens?

Television is full of ads from lawyers wanting to sue pharmaceutical companies. Diabetic medicine harms your heart; Darvon, a mild pain medicine, harms you, even though tons of it have been consumed over the past two to three decades; acne medicine is bad for you, and so on.

A newspaper article cited a case in which RGM Construction sued Tribble and Stephens for a $12,000 unpaid debt. RGM lost on appeal, and the jury was to decide how much RGM should pay the attorneys for Tribble and Stephens. The case had been litigated for nine years, and the attorneys for Tribble and Stephens wanted $1.5 million. The jury awarded them $150,000. RGM had paid their attorneys $500,000. Nine years and over a half million dollars over a $12,000 debt! Everyone's insurance rates will go up, as in medical malpractice. We are not a nation of laws but a nation of lawyers.

In Texas, students entering college are required to be vaccinated against meningitis before entering college. The shot costs $139 at CVS Pharmacy. Why so much if so many doses of the vaccine are to be sold? Much of this cost, most likely, is liability insurance, even if the pharmaceutical company self-insures. A few years ago, there were only a few companies making vaccines because of the liability of a bankrupting class-action lawsuit.

Now malpractice premiums are not the largest expense of health care. Defensive medicine, which has morphed into the maximization of income by doctors and hospitals, is even larger.

Doctors

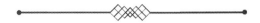

Doctors are responsible for most health-care costs. They see patients, operate on patients, admit patients to hospitals, order tests and diagnostic procedures, and order drugs.

Today neither the doctor nor the patient is concerned with cost because they think that someone else is paying for it. As stated before, the government probably wants increased costs in order to wreck the health-care system, making us ready for government medicine and one world order.

In days gone by, when most of the doctors were good ol' boys until the government shut them down, the medical societies had grievance committees. No doctor wanted to go before his peers because he was accused of overcharging his patients or accused of doing unnecessary surgery. Years ago, at a large hospital, a committee of staff doctors reprimanded a cardiologist and a neurologist for consulting each other on all of their patients. All the cardiologist's patients had headaches, and all the neurologist's patients had chest pain. This would never happen today; every patient has multiple doctors.

The bureaucrats decided that doctors made too much money, even though many doctors worked or were on call most of the time. As the bureaucrats were taught at the Harvard Business School, the way to lower the price is to increase the supply. Foreign medical graduates descended upon us as a cloud of locusts of biblical proportion. As of the publication of this book, 30 percent of our doctors are Indians; a total of 40 percent are foreign medical graduates. As the bureaucrats had been taught, the price came down—but the cost went up. Now, instead of a patient having one doctor, he may have ten.

Some of the best doctors are foreign medical graduates. Many foreign medical graduates have come to the land of milk and honey, but we have some homegrown doctor thieves that can put the best of them to shame.

At one long-term acute-care hospital, each patient has three to ten doctors. Is this thorough, defensive medicine, or is it designed to maximize income? Most of the doctors are foreign medical graduates. Many of the patients have dementia, are unaware of their surroundings, and are vegetating on a ventilator, costing the taxpayers much money.

Two doctors were sent to "Club Fed," minimum-security federal prison, for wheelchair fraud. The doctors ordered motorized wheelchairs for patients who did not need them and probably did not get them. The Nigerian who had put together the scam fled to Nigeria with $9 million.

A general surgeon's employee said that her friend had been to her gynecologist, who sent her to a proctologist downstairs who wanted to operate on her hemorrhoids in a few days. The surgeon asked the employee to ask her friend to come in for a free consultation when he was told that the patient's hemorrhoids did not protrude, bleed, or cause pain. The patient had only minimal hemorrhoids. Some might consider this a normal amount of hemorrhoids.

One could be assured that the proctologist would see a patient whose womb was falling out and needed to see the gynecologist upstairs. These fellows should have been put in jail.

These doctors can get by with some of this hospital thievery under the guise of defensive medicine. In the past, some privately owned hospitals would have an annual golf tournament for the administrative and medical staff. Now, at one small long-term acute-care hospital, they have a cricket match.

At another small hospital, in the doctor's lounge, the TV must have two hundred channels. One could watch a cricket match, a sitcom in Hindi from India, four Spanish stations, or an overweight man who appears to have been shot between the eyes with a red paintball, sitting on the floor chanting in a foreign tongue with foreign subtitles.

Pathologists charge for interpreting laboratory tests done in a hospital. The pathologists say that this is for overseeing the lab. An endocrinologist sends a bill for interpreting a thyroid test. The results for such a test are either normal, too high, or too low.

If patients had to pay directly for their health care, things might be different. The following is a hypothetical letter to a patient's doctor:

When I called you and told you that I had appendicitis, you told me to go to the hospital emergency room. This I did. After waiting for two to three hours, I was put into a room where a Vietnamese lady doctor examined me and ordered some lab work. After another hour or so, the lab work results were given to the ER doctor, who called a surgeon. The surgeon ordered a CT scan of the abdomen and a separate CT scan of the pelvis. Why didn't they just do a CT scan where I hurt rather than two CT scans with two bills?

The emergency room charge was $3,000, and the ER doctor charged me $700. The CT scans were $3,000 apiece, and the radiologist charged me $600 to interpret each CT scan.

Why did I need two CT scans? Even I knew that I had appendicitis after looking up my symptoms on WebMD. Why didn't you just send me to the surgeon's office?

By the time the CT scans were done and the report came back from the radiologist, who was at home or in Hawaii or some other place that had a fax machine, it was past midnight.

I was put in a hospital bed. The surgeon was to see me early in the morning, which was only a few hours away. Were these two expensive CT scans done so the surgeon would not have to come out at night and remove my appendix?

My appendix had leaked, but it was walled off. An infectious disease specialist came by to see me. He charged me $500 for a consultation and $200 a day to come by and say hello. Didn't the surgeon know what kind of antibiotics to give me?

I wasn't having much pain, but a pain specialist came by to see me. He charged me $500 for a consultation and $200 a day to come by and say hello. Doesn't a surgeon who has operated on thousands of patients know what kind of pain medicine to give me?

I had a few extra heartbeats during surgery and in the recovery room. The surgeon called a cardiologist to see me. He charged me $500 for a consultation and $200 a day to come by and say hello to me. Can't the surgeon read an ECG?

There was a small area of my lung that did not expand. They called it atelectasis. A pulmonologist came by to see me. He charged me $500 for a consultation and $200 a day to come by and say hello. It would have been much cheaper if you had just told me to cough.

My blood pressure was slightly elevated. You sent an internal medicine specialist by to see me. He charged me $500 for a consultation and $200 a day to come by and say hello to me. Couldn't you have just given me a blood pressure pill?

My blood sugar was slightly elevated, as it was in the office. An endocrinologist came by to see me. He charged me $500 for a consultation and $200 a day to come by and say hello. Couldn't you or the surgeon have just put me on an insulin sliding scale?

One of my legs hurt. A hematologist came by to see if I needed a blood thinner. He charged me $500 for a consultation and $200 a day to come by and say hello. Couldn't you or the surgeon order a Doppler scan on my veins?

You admitted me to the hospital and came by every day to say hello. You sent me a bill for admission and daily visits, but you did not do anything.

It would have been cheaper if you had sent me to the surgeon's office. He could have admitted me to the hospital and removed my appendix.

Here is the doctor's hypothetical reply:

Dear patient,

It was late, and the surgeon's staff did not want to stay over and wait for you. Many patients would not go straight to the surgeon's office. They might go home first or go eat a pizza.

All the consultants were called because if you sued us, your lawyer would tell the jury that a consultant should have been called.

This is an extreme example. Some degree of this happens with most patients, especially in long-term acute-care hospitals—hospitals where patients go after they have been discharged from a regular hospital. When one has multiple doctors, one gets multiple drugs. In long-term acute-care hospitals, a patient may receive a dozen or more drugs.

Some doctors own hospitals. Some doctors get paid to put patients in hospitals.

Continuing Medical Education (CME)

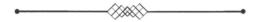

Those who can, do; those who can't, teach.

The state has decreed that health-care providers, formerly known as doctors, must have a certain number of continuing medical education hours yearly to maintain a license to practice medicine. These hours of CME can be obtained by attending meetings, taking computer courses, or receiving in the mail a magazine containing articles, with questions at the end to be answered and mailed back to the sender along with a check for $65. If this is not a scam, the doctor will receive credit for CME hours. What a racket!

Health-care providers, doctors and nurses, must take a course every two years on advanced cardiac life support. This year it is thirty chest compressions and two breaths; two years ago it was fifteen compressions and two breaths.

If one is a specialist, further education is required. Some hospitals require surgeons covering their emergency rooms to have taken and passed a course on advanced trauma life support, established by the American College of Surgeons Committee on Trauma. Who are these dudes on this committee that tell all surgeons in the country what they need to know, who should teach them, where they should take the course, when they should take the course, what questions should be on the test that the doctor must pass in order to make a living, and, above all, how much the doctor must pay for all this?

If one is required to buy something (e.g., a course) in order to make a living, one is at the mercy of the seller.

A surgeon needed an ATLS card to work locum tenens at a hospital. To get this card, one must take a course and pass a test, most likely prepared by dog-and-frog doctors at a medical school rather than by doctors out working in the trenches.

The hapless doctor failed the test; he didn't know how to take care of a stab wound to the heart, even though he had successfully operated on two such cases—probably two more than the teachers of the course. Operating on a stab wound to the heart does not require the skills of Sir Lancelot; the intern could do it. One must open the chest and then open the pericardium—an inelastic covering of the heart containing a few drops of fluid—until the stab wound fills the space between the pericardium and the heart with blood, compressing the heart and reducing the cardiac output.

If care is not taken, when the surgeon opens the pericardium, blood from the small hole in the heart—if the hole were large, the patient would not have made it to the hospital—will hit the surgeon in the face, requiring the circulating nurse to clean his glasses and delicately malposition them back on the surgeon's nose; all the while, the surgeon holds his finger over the hole in the heart. The operation is the surgeon then suturing under his finger with a large silk suture. The pericardium is loosely closed to allow egress of any remaining blood, and a chest tube is put in the chest. Voilà! Another medical miracle. If the patient dies, the plaintiff lawyer will allege that too much time was wasted on a tetanus shot.

The hapless doctor in this case failed because the angry, scornful, militant nurse, reading from her cookbook prepared by the dudes at the American College of Surgeons, said that before going to the operating room, the patient should have a tetanus shot and that the ABCs should be evaluated: *A* is for *airway*, *B* is for *breathing*, and *C* is for *circulation*.

If the patient's blood pressure is low, he will need a large needle put into the pericardium to remove some of the blood on the way to the operating room; the tetanus shot can come the following day.

An angry nurse can deny a doctor his livelihood; his wife will have to stop sitting around the house all day drinking white wine and working crossword puzzles, his kids will have to get a college loan, and he won't be able to buy the latest megadriver for his golf bag—all over a tetanus shot.

The doctor was able to pass by looking at another case.

Lately nurses don't like doctors. "Disdain" and "scorn" might better describe nurses' feelings. Is it because doctors have become more money grubbing, caring more for money than their patients? Is it because of the influx of foreign doctors? Is it because we now have nurse practitioners (nurse doctors)? It was said at a medical meeting that the insurance cartel eventually wants all primary care done by nurses, erroneously thinking that this will save them money.

The government does not think it a monopolistic restraint of trade for a doctor, in order to work, to have to take a course and pass a test concocted by one organization telling the doctor when and where it will take place, how long it will be, and how much it costs.

The late Milton Friedman, a free-market economist, thought that a medical license should not be required to practice medicine; then patients would read the diplomas on the wall. This may be an extreme, but look at what we have now.

Is it because most entering medical school are nerds, devoid of people skills? But people skills don't matter, because when the students finish training, they will be employed by a faceless, impersonal corporation.

The lazy professors just add the college grade score to the MCAT score to decide who will be our doctors, known as health-care providers. Perhaps there are African American patients who would feel more comfortable talking to an African American doctor and Hispanic patients who would feel more comfortable talking to a Hispanic doctor. These people are smart but excel at things other than taking a written test.

Pharmacy

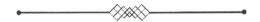

Why is getting a prescription filled such a hassle? It requires only pouring pills from a large bottle into a small bottle. Not exactly. The pharmacist first must determine that the medicine that the doctor prescribed won't harm the patient. The pharmacist must then fill out the label for the bottle of pills, and two or three pages of legal disclaimers must be attached, all to be explained to the patient by the pharmacist if the patient has a question. Pharmacies now sell immunization injections. Now a pharmacist must be a nurse and give the customer a shot.

New Devices and Drugs

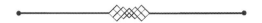

Many years ago, there were few medicinal drugs available. Morphine, digitalis, and phenobarbital are some. An old lady in England found that if one chewed the leaf of a plant, her dropsy (heart failure) improved.

In 1936, Dr. Fleming left the top off an agar plate of bacteria. When some mold (fungus) from another culture blew over to his bacteria plate and killed the bacteria, penicillin was discovered.

During World War I, there was an influenza epidemic. In many cases, the flu was followed by pneumococcal pneumonia, which killed many of the soldiers. A small dose of penicillin would have saved many of these people. Penicillin was truly a wonder drug. It killed many of the bacterial strains. Over the years, many bacteria became resistant to penicillin. More and better antibiotics were discovered. Today there are many antibiotics, some very expensive. A pharmaceutical company may spend $1 billion and ten years developing a drug, and they have to get this money back.

The staphylococcus that causes boils has become resistant to most drugs, including methicillin, a newer penicillin, and must be treated with vancomycin, a drug that must be given intravenously. The blood level of vancomycin must be checked twice daily. If the blood level is too high, it is toxic. If the blood level is too low, it is ineffective. This is very expensive.

Newer antibiotics have been and are being developed. They are and they will be more expensive.

Anticancer drugs can be very expensive. Some oncologists are quitting; they cannot make a living because of the disparity between the reimbursements and the cost of the anticancer drugs. There are now large state and national anticancer (oncology) companies. Anticancer drugs are cheaper when bought by the truckload. It depends on whether one wants to know one's doctor or have a generic company doctor who may or may not speak one's language.

In Houston, a truckload of anticancer drugs was hijacked. The crooks, along with the old gentleman who was supposed to "fence" the drugs, were arrested. The thieves were also charged with kidnapping, because they made the driver drive the truck. In Texas, no crime is beyond one's imagination.

There are many expensive diagnostic modalities: CT scans, MRI scans, angiograms, and so on. If the doctors own the CT machine or MRI scanner or get paid for reading the results of the study, the machines may or may not be overutilized. A computerized tomography (CT) scan shows an x-ray of a slice through the body. A magnetic resonance imaging (MRI) scan uses a magnet and is better than a CT scan for some things. Brain tumors are one example.

A lithotripter is a machine where one is put in a tub of water and shock waves are used to break up kidney stones in order for the stone fragments to become small enough to pass, avoiding an open operation.

Today the treatment of a heart attack may be to go directly to the cath lab, have the clot dissolved, have the artery opened with a balloon, and have a stent put in the diseased artery. A basket can now be put into the coronary artery to remove a clot.

Laparoscopic surgery requires expensive equipment, but the shorter hospital stay and the shorter convalescent period makes it a plus for saving money, not to mention less pain and less time away from work.

Hyperbaric oxygen treatment is now being used to treat several conditions. Hemoglobin in the red blood cells combines with oxygen in the lungs to form oxyhemoglobin. When the red blood cells reach the tissues in the body, the oxygen is released to the cells. Because the hemoglobin is almost completely saturated with oxygen, to get a high saturation of oxygen in the tissue, 100 percent oxygen under pressure is used to dissolve oxygen in the blood serum. To achieve this, the patient is put in a Plexiglas chamber and 100 percent oxygen is pumped in under pressure. There are chambers that hold one patient, and there are chambers that hold a dozen. In the multiperson chamber, a plastic hood that fits over the patient's head and is snug around the neck has 100 percent oxygen pumped in to it. The chamber itself contains air under pressure. A nurse without an oxygen hood accompanies the patients.

The hyperbaric oxygen chamber is used to treat carbon monoxide poisoning. One exhales carbon dioxide—CO_2, one carbon atom and two oxygen atoms. Carbon monoxide has one carbon atom and one oxygen atom. Carbon monoxide has a much greater affinity for oxygen than does hemoglobin. Carbon monoxide is formed when there is not enough oxygen for an oxygen atom to join the carbon; the use of a space heater in a closed space can cause this. Hyperbaric oxygen oxygenates the hemoglobin and hastens the elimination of the carbon monoxide by furnishing an oxygen atom. The oxygen dissolved in the plasma sustains life in the meantime.

When Bill O'Reilly, on his show, asked Joe Namath if he had brain injury from playing professional football, Joe said, "Yes, but it was corrected by hyperbaric oxygen treatment," and showed before-and-after MRI scans of his brain.

If this is valid, a study should be done. Joe probably has good genes, because when they dragged out some retired NFL players at an NFL game, Joe appeared younger than most, although he was older.

The bends are caused by nitrogen bubbling out of the blood and into the tissues. The amount of nitrogen in the tissue is a function of depth and time. Some caisson workers digging tunnels were under air pressure for a shift; when the workers came out, they developed the bends, also called caisson disease. Some offshore oil rigs have a hyperbaric chamber on the platform to treat commercial divers.

When a patient is put in a single hyperbaric chamber and compressed to two atmospheric pressures (we are already at one atmosphere of pressure), the patient might complain of being hot because, according to Charles's law, when a gas is compressed, the heat of the gas increases. If the rate of compression is slowed, there appears to be less heat, or the heat dissipates.

A diesel engine works on this principle; the compressed hot air ignites the diesel fuel. A refrigerator does the opposite; the gas expands and cools.

Charles's law is related to the Deflategate controversy of 2015, which began when the Indianapolis Colts accused the New England Patriots of letting the air out of their footballs, making them easier for Tom Brady to throw. No mention was made as to whether the Indianapolis Colts put air into their footballs. Mr. Kraft, the owner of the New England Patriots, was fined $1 million, and Tom Brady was suspended for the first four games of the season.

The dude running the NFL who levied these fines had apparently never heard of Charles's law. The pump used to inflate the footballs contained hot air. The faster that the football was inflated, the hotter the air in the football. The temperature inside was seventy-five degrees; the temperature outside was seventeen degrees. Dude, the hot air in the football cooled, thus decreasing the pressure in the football. Why wasn't an experiment done by inflating a football in a seventy-five-degree room and taking it outside in the seventeen-degree temperature?

Today there are stroke centers, usually in large hospitals where a neurologist is available, where one's chances for survival and having less brain damage are enhanced because of the new treatments and the experts knowing how to apply them.

If one has a stroke, it is important to have treatment started within two hours. If Granny has a stroke, don't call an ambulance; put her in a car and drive her to the stroke center, where a wire basket can be put into an artery and threaded into the brain to remove a blood clot, and a clot dissolving drug can be given, possibly limiting the amount of brain damage.

A man returned from a scuba-diving trip in Mexico. He was paralyzed and could not get off the plane. He had the bends. A rapid trip to a hyperbaric oxygen chamber relieved his paralysis by forcing the nitrogen bubbles back into the blood.

The patient might have scuba dived the day that he boarded the plane. Instead of being at the surface, he kept going up another eight thousand feet, the usual cabin pressure of an airliner. The patient might have scuba dived several days in a row, or two or three times a day. The navy has diving tables showing how much longer one needs to spend ascending on a dive because of residual nitrogen in the tissue from previous recent dives. Most likely, this patient did not consult the navy diving tables.

Hyperbaric oxygen is used to treat refractory osteomyelitis, refractory diabetic foot ulcers, radiation necrosis (bone damage from radiation cancer treatment), and skin flaps that appear in jeopardy because of decreased blood supply as a result of an operation.

Today, especially in long-term acute-care hospitals, patients receive physical therapy to strengthen their muscles. The patients also receive occupational therapy to help them take care of their daily needs.

One can no longer die at home. One has to die in a hospital, a long-term acute-care hospital, or in a hospice.

Most of these people have an intravenous line, most likely a central line—a catheter threaded into the vena cava. Today most central lines are percutaneous indwelling central catheter (PICC) lines. Using an ultrasound to locate the vein in the upper arm, a technician threads a catheter into the vena cava. An x-ray is taken to check the position of the catheter. A house doctor may be called to look at the catheter's position on the x-ray in order for the catheter to be used until the radiologist can read the x-ray and dictate a report, or put the report in a computer.

The technician can see that the catheter is well placed. Cut the house doctor and the radiologist out of the loop and save money. Perhaps a metal-tipped catheter that would show on an ultrasound could be used, eliminating the x-ray technician also.

The Food and Drug Administration (FDA) is responsible for seeing that we have safe food and drugs. Many years ago, thalidomide, a sleeping pill, caused babies to be born without limbs if their mothers took the drug during pregnancy. This disaster, along with bankrupting class-action lawsuits against pharmaceutical companies, has made the FDA so careful that few new drugs can come to market. Only eleven new drugs were approved in one year, although many more were discovered. Now it takes ten years and $1 billion dollars to bring a new drug to market. The FDA is almost incapacitated. Patients die and go blind waiting on approval of drugs by the FDA.

EnteroVioform, a great drug for avoiding "turistas" when traveling in Mexico or in other countries in which one is likely to get diarrhea, was removed from the market after many years of use. It is rumored that three Japanese citizens had neuritis after taking the drug.

Darvon, a mild painkiller, was taken off the market recently because it allegedly damages one's heart.

Turn on the TV and it seems that all the ads are from lawyers. Avendia, a diabetes medicine, harms one's heart. Acne medicine harms one's bowels. The list goes on.

One would think that if a pharmaceutical company spent ten years and a billion dollars developing a drug and didn't lie about the studies and the drug was approved by the FDA, people should be barred from suing them.

Erbitux, an anticancer drug, was turned down, not approved, by the FDA. Sam, the president of the company, dumped his stock. Pete, Martha Stewart's stock broker, phoned her and told her that there was a rumor on the floor that Sam was selling his stock. Martha told Pete to sell hers because they planned to sell it anyway when the stock reached sixty dollars per share.

The US government prosecuted Martha and Pete and sent them to jail for lying, although there is no way that the government could know whether or not Martha and

Pete planned to sell her stock when it reached sixty dollars per share.

At trial, the judge would not allow the jury to be told that Martha Stewart was not being charged with insider trading. Most juries have the mental capacity of eighth graders.

Our country has degenerated into a police state. When the government wants to put you in jail, they put you in jail. Look what was done to John Edwards. Roger Clemens was tried on "evidence" stored in a beer can for six years. The person who had dominion and control over the evidence was a known liar who, most likely, in my opinion, was helping the government hang Roger Clemens for the government's granting him immunity.

Martha Stewart was convicted for being "irascible."

The FDA changed their minds and approved Erbitux.

Who are these dudes at the FDA? Some or many come from institutions that test drugs for pharmaceutical companies. If the drug is approved, the pharmaceutical company no longer will have to pay to have the drug tested. Only eleven drugs were approved by the FDA in one year. More testing means more money for the testers.

Fraud

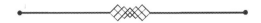

What is fraud? Obviously, charging the government or the insurance companies for services or things not delivered is fraud. Is delivering services that may or may not be needed fraud? Or is that being thorough? Is calling your friends, who will call you as a consultant, fraud? Or is that being thorough and protecting yourself from lawsuits? Is admitting a patient to a hospital that you own in part fraud? Or is that being careful? Is ordering a wheelchair for a patient fraud if the doctor gets a kickback from the wheelchair company? It certainly is—especially if the wheelchair is not delivered.

Two doctors were sentenced to "Club Fed"—minimum-security federal prison—for wheelchair fraud. The doctors were paid for ordering motorized wheelchairs that weren't delivered. The doctors went to jail. The Nigerian who put the deal together fled to Nigeria with $9 million. Some of these Nigerians have come to the Land of Milk and Honey. It's so easy.

A doctor inherited a forty-year-old patient with cerebral palsy whose devoted mother had taken excellent care of him for years. The doctor was called by a medical supply company that asked if he would sign for a large number of items for this patient. The doctor said that he would sign the order, but he first called the mother, who said that her son's nonmotorized wheelchair was worn out and that he needed another. Had the doctor signed the order, the government would have been charged thousands of dollars for undelivered items. There is a chance that someone else signed the order or the doctor's name was forged.

Home health lends itself to thievery. A number of years ago, a man and his nurse wife started a home health company. The company was so successful that the man flew his friends to football games in the company jet. The company remained successful until the man was put in jail for fraud. He should have fled to Nigeria. Then again, jail might be better than Nigeria.

South Florida generates much fraud. Perhaps this is because of the large population of Medicare recipients there. There are so many legitimate Medicare claims that it may be difficult to pick out the fraudulent ones.

Is it fraud for the emergency room doctors to order too many CT scans, x-rays, and labs to keep the hospital from replacing them with another ER group? Is it fraud to overutilize if you own the place? Is it overutilization, being thorough, or trying to keep from being sued?

How can the system keep from paying for unnecessary labs, x-rays, and consultants? Even honest, competent doctors don't want to be sued.

Scooters for old people are lined up in front of a pawn shop a few blocks from a hospital.

Closer watch should be kept on the taxpayers' money.

Conclusion

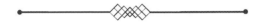

One of Professor C. Northcote Parkinson's economic laws is "bureaucrats make work for each other." He further states that a bureaucracy is death of any achievement."

John Stossel outlined the laws, permits, and regulations with which he would have to comply in order to open a lemonade stand in Manhattan. What if Mr. Stossel wanted to add to his enterprise a first-aid station manned by a nurse, similar to a school nurse? Would an environmental impact study be required? Would the nurse have to show that she'd had diversity and sensitivity training? Would there have to be three pages of clinical trial studies and legal disclaimers accompanying every aspirin tablet?

Think of all the laws, rules, and regulations that you can and put an exponent above your list; you will then have an idea of what hospitals endure.

In addition to the bureaucrats' rules and regulations, hospitals need expensive defensive measures, because under every rock, waiting to sue them, is a lawyer.

The propaganda ministry (ABC, CBS, NBC, the *New York Times*, etc.) kept the masses confused by convincing them that the health-care problems were caused by a few bad doctors, and all that was needed to fix the problem was to get rid of these bad apples.

If we have government-controlled medicine, the insurance oligarchs will still administer it. Ross Perot became a billionaire in part because he owned the National Heritage Health Insurance Company, which administered Medicaid in Texas. The CEO of UnitedHealthcare, which administered Texas Medicaid HMO Evercare (dubbed "Nevercare" by the doctors), had $1.7 billion in unexercised stock options. Some of Warren Buffet's wealth came from owning insurance companies. Did these insurance companies do business with the government, as did UnitedHealthcare and National Heritage Insurance Company?

To fix our sick health-care system, we were given Obamacare medicine, which turned out to be worse than the disease.

People in the United States are in the following categories:

Medicare	47 million	15%
Employer insurance	150 million	48%
Medicaid/CHIP	40 million	13%
Uninsured	50 million	16%

The propagandist would have the populace believe that people with cancer and babies were dying in the streets for lack of medical care, as are the marasmic people dying in the streets of Rangoon.

With the destruction of the private health-care system, we would eventually get one-payer health care, the dream of the socialists and the one-worlders, and a windfall for the insurance cartel that would administer it.

One-payer health care would be very inefficient if run by the government (think VA) and would endure much stealing if run by insurance companies.

The government is concerned with overutilization. Who will decide what overutilization is? In days when the doctors were a bunch of good ol' boys, the hospital staff committees would address the problem; today it will be the US government.

Obamacare has cut back on Medicare funding, including what doctors are being paid to treat Medicare patients. The doctors will outfox them; each patient will have four doctors seeing him or her instead of three, or five instead of four, or six instead of five.

Obamacare has so many programs that there will be more bureaucrats and government workers administering the programs than there are doctors:

- community health
- early retiree insurance plans
- in-home long-term health
- Community Living Assistance Service and Support (CLASS)
- nutrition in restaurants
- prevention counselling in Medicare
- employer-based personal wellness reward programs

- prevention as a guaranteed "Essential Health Benefit"
- accountable care organizations
- Independent at Home

Who knows what is in the thousand or so other pages? We will have legions of government bureaucrats and workers trying to micromanage everyone's health care. This can only be expensive and most inefficient, to the detriment of all.

What Can Be Done—Efficiency

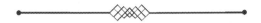

When individuals are free to innovate and are rewarded for doing so, everyone benefits; when a pervasive government controls everything, the result will be stagnation. This has been proven over and over again, but people still want the government to control everything and everybody—Obamacare.

If everyone is entitled to health care, which everyone already has, then health care, or basic health care, should be defined. Is health care a private room with a flat screen TV and a nurse giving the patient IV narcotics every four hours? In some cases, that's what we have today.

The companies that buy insurance for 48 percent of the population should be allowed to deal directly with doctors, clinics, and hospitals rather than insurance companies, unless the company thinks it better to deal with an insurance company.

If doctors were paid immediately and did not have to hire an extra employee to get permission from the insurance company, sometimes hanging on the phone for an hour, the cost of the doctor's services could be reduced.

If a company wants to use an insurance company, the company or corporation should be able to buy insurance from any insurance company in the country or in the world, rather than from the two or three insurance companies allowed to do business in the state.

Was it Sir John Anton who said, "Absolute power corrupts absolutely"? If an employee could get insurance only through the company, the company might hire cheap doctors, "warm bodies in white coats," thinking that money was being saved. Employees should be able to buy their own insurance or see their own doctors. The company could pay part, and the employees could pay the difference. Of course, the company would have to make sure that the employees' doctors were not ripping them off.

The insurance cartel has had absolute power. Look what they and their lackey lawyers have done.

When the US government has absolute power (Obamacare) over our health care, what do you think will happen?

An argument for government medicine is that we are the only civilized country without government medicine. We are, or perhaps were, the country with the most freedom to start a business.

In Great Britain, the rich go to the private doctors who treat the rich Arabs.

A surgeon in the United States went to Israel and gave a professor $5,000 to remove his mother's gall bladder, avoiding a wait and avoiding a second-year resident removing his mother's gall bladder. We are all equal, only some are more equal than others.

With Medicare and Medicaid, the "fiddler doctrine" should be instituted. He who pays the fiddler calls the tune. Waste and fraud should be eliminated. Some think that the government does not want to eliminate fraud, making us ready for government medicine.

Today, because of advanced directives, resuscitation is attempted on ninety-plus-year-old patients with dementia. A ninety-four-year-old patient with dementia, on a ventilator, is a "full code," meaning that when the patient dies, the nurses will pound on her chest and give her injections of epinephrine, all to no avail. This is done if the family does not sign a do-not-resuscitate directive. This is all right with the hospital, because the hospital will bill Medicare for this futile attempt at resurrection.

A nurse in a nursing home called 911 to have the emergency crew come resuscitate a patient—more likely resurrect a patient. The nursing home may face criminal charges because this is the nursing home's policy. One's heart cannot remain stopped for over five minutes without brain or heart damage, unless it is a child who drowned in cold water.

Now not only can one no longer die in a hospital without a futile and expensive attempt at resuscitation; the same is the case in a nursing home.

Quit trying to resuscitate ninety-plus-year-old patients with dementia when they die. No one has been resurrected in about 1,980 years.

A study showed that of the last thousand patients ninety years of age or older who had cardiac arrest from asystole (heart stoppage), none were resuscitated. The study could also include PEA (pulseless electrical activity) and bradycardia (heart slowing). The study could be presented (not that they need it) to a panel of the country's leading doctors, who could recommend no resuscitative efforts be made on some patients. This could prevent attacks on the doctors by lawyers. The government could refuse payment unless other circumstances were documented.

The payer of the bills might ask why patients vegetating on ventilators during the last two weeks of their lives need six doctors to come by every day and send a bill. How many patients in long-term acute-care hospitals who have cardiac resuscitation (code) leave the hospital alive?

Patients without insurance should pay hospitals the same as insurance companies pay hospitals, not four to five times as much. Patients with no resources could go to a charity or teaching hospital, where the care, in most instances, would be better than the care in private hospitals with private doctors. There are just no frills. If the private hospitals did not pad their bills and rob patients, people with limited resources could afford to go to private hospitals rather than to charity hospitals.

The Emergency Medical Treatment and Active Labor Act (EMTALA) should be repealed. This bill allows Medicaid patients to go to hospital emergency rooms rather than to doctors' offices, costing the taxpayers five or more times as much as a doctor visit. The Medicaid patient can call an ambulance instead of a taxi.

The government plans a pilot program to give money to the hospital to take care of a patient. The hospital would pay the doctors and buy the drugs and supplies. This would take care of patients having six doctors. With accountants running things, the patients would be slighted.

This has been tried before with the Independent Physicians Association, where the doctors were paid to "keep the patients well." The doctors kept the money and neglected the patient they had been paid to take care of.

The government is more interested in controlling people than in their well-being; and to have the insurance and hospital oligarch get richer, sharing some of their lucre with the politicians.

Allegedly forty veterans died waiting to be seen at a VA hospital. A professor said that the VA hospital was always full because the patients did not want to go home, the families did not want the patients to come home, the hospital did not want the patients to go home because without a full hospital their budget would be cut, and the doctors want the patient to remain in the hospital because when a new patient arrived, the doctor would have to work him up.

At a VA hospital, six cataract operations are done by 3:00 p.m. At a surgical center, twelve to sixteen cataract operations are done by 1:00 p.m. Residents are operating at the VA hospital. Some say, "Get more doctors at the VA." It would not solve the problem if the doctors didn't work.

If a doctor is paid the same whether he does one

operation or ten operations a day, he is not going to start early and stay late. Because their incomes are capped, Canadian doctors work less. The wealth of a nation is the sum of that which is produced. If there is a disincentive for people to work, through government regulations and taxes, the nation will be less wealthy. This may not be true in the United States; we just print the money.

A cure for diabetes would be a great boon to society. In the meanwhile, education appears to be the only solution—exercise and don't get fat.

The Patient's Pain Bill of Rights should be repealed. It has given us a new class of junkies.

Advanced directives should be modified. This gives unknowing, uncaring family members the right to make medical decisions, costing the taxpayers much money.

Call off the insurance oligarchs and their lackey lawyers by way of tort reform. States are doing this now.

Call off the propagandists and phrasemongers who bash doctors. Have them direct their efforts to health: eat right, don't get fat, exercise, and don't do drugs. Pharmacies are now selling vaccinations. Soon the pharmacies will sell health care, if the government doesn't stop them. We will have CVSCare and WalmartCare.

Church-named hospitals, even though they make an enormous amount of money, need to take an occasional charity patient, either to maintain their tax-exempt status or to look good and help.

Church-named hospitals pay no taxes. Private and stock exchange hospitals do, giving the church-named hospitals an advantage. One might think that tax-exempt hospitals would provide cheaper care, but this does not seem to be the case. Do these profits go to building churches and to paying preachers?

The 16 percent of uninsured people in the United States may be healthy and need no insurance, or they may wish to go to a charity institution if needed. The charity hospitals staffed by interns and residents, and supervised by medical school professors, usually provide better care than private hospitals and private doctors.

Telemedicine

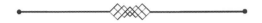

Telemedicine is a patient sending the doctor his or her picture and results of studies, instead of the doctor seeing the patient in person and laying hands on that patient.

Telemedicine may be used to advantage for patients far from a medical facility, or perhaps to follow-up with a dermatologist or send a selfie of a patient's post-op hernia incision.

Some long-term acute-care hospitals are replacing their house doctors with telemedicine. Will the nurse send a picture of the patient with the pertinent studies to a doctor in Boston? We already have telemedicine; the nurse calls the doctor. This sounds like more stealing.

Today, long-term acute-care hospitals are replacing house doctors with teledoctors, who have never seen the patients before. We already have teledoctors; the nurse calls the patient's doctor to ask about the patient.

Today, long-term acute-care hospitals will have one teledoctor instead of ten house doctors. Today the nurse will call the teledoctor, generating a bill to Medicare, instead of calling the patient's doctor, because the nurse has to call the answering service of the attending physician.

The attending physician may take awhile to answer his or her page, or may not answer at all.

When the attending physician answers the call, he or she may tell the nurse to call one of the other five to six doctors who see the patient daily and send a bill.

The nurses may be encouraged to call the teledoctor first because it is a new income stream for the hospital.

In the past, treating patients over the telephone was a malpractice hazard.

A few wrongful death lawsuits because a patient died without a doctor putting his or her hands on the patient may cause reevaluation of telemedicine.

When Medicare gets the bills for all these phone calls, Medicare may take a look at telemedicine.

Continuing medical education (CME) sounds good; it implies that it will make our doctors smart. CME has generated a new industry. Doctors and nurses are required to take a course, acute cardiac life support (ALCS), every two years. There is nothing really new being taught in this course. If there were an earth-shaking change, a memo could be sent out.

Most doctors have narrowed their fields, but the Texas board requires, in addition to CME, that doctors have an hour of "ethics," which could be taught on blood transfusions and Jehovah's Witnesses, dementia, and so on.

Doctors can read books and journals; they don't need bureaucrats telling them to spend their time and money on useless endeavors.

Do away with CME!

What can be done?

- Obamacare can be replaced with no care.
- People who want to buy insurance can buy insurance from any company in the country.
- People on Medicare and Medicaid are covered.
- People who have insurance through their jobs are covered.
- People who do not fall into the above categories can go to an eleemosynary (charity) institution.

Hospitals aren't interested in controlling costs; they make money.

The government has no interest in controlling the cost of health care. The government can't go broke; the government just prints money. Plus, the government is inefficient.

The insurance cartel does not want to control the cost of health care, because the higher the cost, the higher the premiums. The resulting one-payer care will be administered by insurance companies.

Companies that provide health care for employees should be able to deal directly with doctors, clinics, and hospitals, buying insurance only if the company believes it to be the best deal. The employees should have an out if they want to see their own doctors. Of course, the company should make sure that the employee doctor is not ripping them off.

During World War II, Henry J. Kaiser, a California shipbuilder, along with a doctor friend, started Kaiser

Permanente to take care of their employees' needs. Kaiser Permanente has survived as Kaiser Managed Care with 10.2 million members, 186,457 employees, and 18,651 salaried doctors.

Years ago, in Baton Rouge, Louisiana, there was Stanacola, Standard Oil Company of Louisiana, now Exxon, which took care of Exxon employees. The Stanacola doctors were despised by many of the Baton Rouge doctors because of the perceived damage to the private practice of medicine. Stanacola is still here, merged with People's Health Network.

Lawsuits and the fear of lawsuits caused by the insurance cartels and lawyers are the greatest drivers of exorbitant health-care costs. As stated, this is their plan to destroy private medicine. Some states have passed tort-reform legislation, limiting awards for pain and suffering, which controls lawsuits because old retired people receive more medical care and experience more bad outcomes. Because the old patients are no longer employed, there is no economic damage. No good lawyer will handle a case capped at $200,000–$250,000. There are informed consent laws stating the complications of an operation that could happen, precluding lawsuits. Some states have a committee of doctors and lawyers who must review malpractice suits. If the committee said that you were guilty of actionable malpractice, your insurance carrier would want to settle. If the committee said that there was no malpractice, the plaintiff lawyer would not want to go to court with a committee of expert witnesses against him or her. More could be done to curtail lawsuits. Everybody dies—some sooner, some later.

Money is being wasted by allowing six or more doctors daily to see hospital patients. Not only do the consultants send bills for daily visits; they also order tests. Perhaps the payers of these bills should ask why this patient needs all these doctors seeing him or her daily rather than just rendering an opinion. All hospital patients could be taken care of by a hospitalist. Patients may not want a doctor that they cannot understand. The hospital may hire a hospitalist that represents the hospital's interest rather than the interest of the patient. Companies that are paying for their employees' health care might pay attention to their health-care costs.

Hospital costs are the principle costs of health care. The hospitals don't want to lower the cost of health care, because the hospitals make more money and pass their costs to the insurance companies. Those insurance companies are not interested in controlling health-care costs, because higher costs mean higher premiums.

Much of the hospital costs are liability premiums and defensive measures to defend or to prevent lawsuits; however, the enormous hospital bills should be examined. Patients' physical therapy and occupational therapy bills probably could be combined. Automatic lab test costs could be reduced. Hospital bills should be examined.

Lumps and bumps should be removed in a doctor's office rather than in a hospital or in a surgical center. The insurance companies pay very little for an office procedure, but if the insurance paid well for removing a mole in the doctor's office, they would be overwhelmed with claims, because everyone has a skin lesion that could be removed.

Inguinal hernias could be repaired using local anesthesia as an outpatient procedure, using a subcuticular suture to close the skin, even though it may take it a bit longer than skin staples. Rather than returning to the doctor's office, a photo of the incision could be sent to the doctor's office, and the patient could talk to the doctor or to the nurse.

Something should be done about the Food and Drug Administration (FDA), which has been paralyzed by the fiasco regarding Thalidomide, a sleeping pill that caused babies to be born with flippers for limbs when given to pregnant mothers, as well as more bankrupting class-action suits (e.g., IUDs from A. H. Robins and breast implants from Dow Corning). Something should also be done about class action suits in general. If ten years and a billion dollars were spent developing a drug, and the studies were honest, people should be barred from suing.

Something should be done about the high cost of drugs, brought about by excessive studies required to get the drug to market. Allow drugs to be imported. At Larry Mellon's hospital in Haiti, Larry bought Chloromycetin for 1.9 cents a capsule from a Scandinavian country when the Chloromycetin pills sold for 60 cents apiece in the United States.

Call off the phrasemongers and propagandists, the lapdogs of the insurance cartels and their lackey lawyers, who have convinced the populace that the health-care problem is caused by a few bad doctors, failing to explain why some of the best doctors have many lawsuits filed against them.

Those who want the federal government to run our health care should look at the countries that have tried such plans. In England, the rich go to private doctors who treat the rich Arabs; others wait in line unless what they want is not covered (e.g., there is age limit on dialysis). Supposedly, the biggest employer in the world is the Chinese Army; second is the British health-care system.

In Canada, the doctors don't work very much. There is a waiting list. Some patients come to the United States for treatment.

In Scandinavia, people are slim and ride bicycles.

VA hospitals are government health care. Forty veterans died waiting to be seen at VA hospitals.

Currently, 20 percent of Medicare money is spent on diabetes, probably including complications of heart disease, strokes, foot and ankle ulcers, occluded leg arteries, and end-stage renal disease. Of the total number of diabetics, 90 to 95 percent are adult-onset diabetics or non-insulin-dependent diabetes victims; usually these people are overweight. Education should start at an early age; however, it probably would be futile, because people eat as their parents eat. In years past, schools had recess and playgrounds where children could get some exercise. Today there probably would be drug deals and knife fights.

In a Russian state-run auto company, 1.4 million workers make 700,000 cars. In Fiat plants, 130,000 workers make 2.5 million cars. Of course, we are comparing Russian auto workers with Italian auto workers.

Socialism does not work in making automobiles or in providing health care. Look at the post office. Not only are the workers government workers, but they are also union workers. Will the doctors and the nurses be unionized?

In ancient Rome, the masses were kept content by giving them bread and circuses. Today it is McDonalds and the NFL for the masses, who neither know nor care that their health care is being dismantled and that their freedom is being lost.

				Insurance portion computed from information vouched by employer or insurance carrier and may be subject to change	Page No.
			02/21/11		1

------- DETAIL CHARGES -------

Date	Code	Description		Charge	Amount
1/28/10		PRIVATE RHB	1005A	1133.00	1133.00
1/29/10		PRIVATE RHB	1005A	1133.00	1133.00
1/30/10		PRIVATE RHB	1005A	1133.00	1133.00
1/31/10		PRIVATE RHB	1005A	1133.00	1133.00
1/01/10		PRIVATE RHB	1005A	1133.00	1133.00
1/02/10		PRIVATE RHB	1005A	1133.00	1133.00
1/03/10		PRIVATE RHB	1005A	1133.00	1133.00
1/04/10		PRIVATE RHB	1005A	1133.00	1133.00
1/05/10		PRIVATE RHB	1005A	1133.00	1133.00
1/06/10		PRIVATE RHB	1005A	1133.00	1133.00
1/07/10		PRIVATE RHB	1005A	1133.00	1133.00
	TOTAL	PRIVATE RHB		12463.00	12463.00
0/28/10	D0704	RHB FX LOW EXT M<28.15 D0704		.00	
	TOTAL	0024		.00	
0/28/10		FUROSEMIDE 40MG UD TAB		4.00	4.00
0/28/10		WARFARIN 7.5MG UD TAB		9.50	9.50
0/28/10	J1815	INSULIN GLARGINE 100UNIT/ML PEN		222.00	222.00
0/28/10		FLUTICASONE 50MCG NASAL SPR		356.00	356.00
0/28/10		NACL 0.65% NOSE SPRAY 45ML		16.50	16.50
0/28/10		POLYETHYLENE GLYCOL 17GM UD PKT		16.50	16.50
0/28/10	J1815	INSULIN HUMAN REGULAR 3ML VIAL		55.00	55.00
0/28/10	J3490	LABETOLOL 5MG/ML AMP 20ML		29.00	29.00
0/28/10	J2405	ONDANSETRON 4MG INJ		642.00	642.00
		QUANTITY OF	4		
0/28/10		DOCUSATE SODIUM 100MG UD CAP		8.00	8.00
		QUANTITY OF	2		
0/28/10		NIFEDIPINE 30MG SR UD TAB		33.00	33.00
		QUANTITY OF	2		
0/28/10		OMEPRAZOLE 20MG SR UD CAP		64.00	64.00
		QUANTITY OF	2		
0/28/10		POVIDONE IODINE 10% SOL 120ML		10.50	10.50
0/28/10	Q0179	ONDANSETRON 4MG UD TAB		540.00	540.00
		QUANTITY OF	4		
0/28/10		CARVEDILOL 12.5MG UD TAB		16.50	16.50
0/28/10		GUAIFENESIN 600MG LA UD TAB		4.00	4.00
0/29/10		FUROSEMIDE 40MG UD TAB		8.00	8.00
		QUANTITY OF	2		
0/29/10		WARFARIN 7.5MG UD TAB		9.50	9.50
0/29/10		POLYETHYLENE GLYCOL 17GM UD PKT		16.50	16.50
0/29/10		POTASSIUM Cl 20MEQ SR UD TAB		4.50	4.50
0/29/10		DOCUSATE SODIUM 100MG UD CAP		8.00	8.00
		QUANTITY OF	2		
0/29/10		NIFEDIPINE 30MG SR UD TAB		33.00	33.00
		QUANTITY OF	2		
0/29/10		OMEPRAZOLE 20MG SR UD CAP		64.00	64.00
		QUANTITY OF	2		
0/29/10		CARVEDILOL 12.5MG UD TAB		33.00	33.00
		QUANTITY OF	2		

Fees for physician services, consultations and interpretations are billed individually and are not included as part of the hospital invoice.

K0564

02/21/11

PAGE NO
2

Insurance portion computed
from information verified
by employer or insurance
carrier and may be subject
to change

Date	Description	Amount	Amount
1/29/10	GUAIFENESIN 600MG LA UD TAB	8.00	8.00
	QUANTITY OF 2		
1/29/10	HYDROCODONE W/APAP 10/325 UD	17.00	17.00
	QUANTITY OF 2		
1/30/10	FUROSEMIDE 40MG UD TAB	8.00	8.00
	QUANTITY OF 2		
1/30/10	POLYETHYLENE GLYCOL 17GM UD PKT	16.50	16.50
1/30/10	POTASSIUM Cl 20MEQ SR UD TAB	4.50	4.50
1/30/10	DOCUSATE SODIUM 100MG UD CAP	8.00	8.00
	QUANTITY OF 2		
1/30/10	NIFEDIPINE 30MG SR UD TAB	33.00	33.00
	QUANTITY OF 2		
1/30/10	OMEPRAZOLE 20MG SR UD CAP	64.00	64.00
	QUANTITY OF 2		
1/30/10	CARVEDILOL 12.5MG UD TAB	33.00	33.00
	QUANTITY OF 2		
1/30/10	GUAIFENESIN 600MG LA UD TAB	8.00	8.00
	QUANTITY OF 2		
1/30/10	HYDROCODONE W/APAP 10/325 UD	17.00	17.00
	QUANTITY OF 2		
1/31/10	FUROSEMIDE 40MG UD TAB	4.00	4.00
1/31/10	WARFARIN 5MG UD TAB	7.50	7.50
1/31/10	POLYETHYLENE GLYCOL 17GM UD PKT	16.50	16.50
1/31/10	POTASSIUM Cl 20MEQ SR UD TAB	4.50	4.50
1/31/10	KENADERM 60GM OINTMENT	294.00	294.00
1/31/10	DOCUSATE SODIUM 100MG UD CAP	8.00	8.00
	QUANTITY OF 2		
1/31/10	NIFEDIPINE 30MG SR UD TAB	16.50	16.50
1/31/10	OMEPRAZOLE 20MG SR UD CAP	64.00	64.00
	QUANTITY OF 2		
1/31/10	LEVOFLOXACIN 500MG UD TAB	250.50	250.50
	QUANTITY OF 3		
1/31/10	CARVEDILOL 12.5MG UD TAB	33.00	33.00
	QUANTITY OF 2		
1/31/10	GUAIFENESIN 600MG LA UD TAB	8.00	8.00
	QUANTITY OF 2		
1/31/10	HYDROCODONE W/APAP 10/325 UD	17.00	17.00
	QUANTITY OF 2		
./01/10	WARFARIN 4MG TABLET	7.00	7.00
./01/10	HYDROCODONE W/APAP 5/325MG UD	4.50	4.50
./01/10	POLYETHYLENE GLYCOL 17GM UD PKT	16.50	16.50
./01/10	POTASSIUM Cl 20MEQ SR UD TAB	4.50	4.50
./01/10	DOCUSATE SODIUM 100MG UD CAP	8.00	8.00
	QUANTITY OF 2		
./01/10	NIFEDIPINE 30MG SR UD TAB	33.00	33.00
	QUANTITY OF 2		
./01/10	OMEPRAZOLE 20MG SR UD CAP	64.00	64.00
	QUANTITY OF 2		
./01/10	LEVOFLOXACIN 250MG UD TAB	155.00	155.00
	QUANTITY OF 2		
./01/10	LEVOFLOXACIN 500MG UD TAB	83.50-	83.50-
./01/10	CARVEDILOL 12.5MG UD TAB	33.00	33.00
	QUANTITY OF 2		

Fees for physician services, consultations and interpretations are billed
individually and are not included as part of the hospital invoice.

Insurance portion computed from information verified by employer of insurance carrier and may be subject to change

| | | | Statement Date 02/21/11 | | | Page No. 3 |

Date	Code	Description		Amount	Amount	
/01/10		GUAIFENESIN 600MG LA UD TAB		8.00	8.00	
		QUANTITY OF 2				
/02/10		FUROSEMIDE 40MG UD TAB		12.00	12.00	
		QUANTITY OF 3				
/02/10		POLYETHYLENE GLYCOL 17GM UD PKT		16.50	16.50	
/02/10		POTASSIUM CL 20MEQ SR UD TAB		4.50	4.50	
/02/10		DOCUSATE SODIUM 100MG UD CAP		8.00	8.00	
		QUANTITY OF 2				
/02/10		NIFEDIPINE 30MG SR UD TAB		33.00	33.00	
		QUANTITY OF 2				
/02/10		OMEPRAZOLE 20MG SR UD CAP		64.00	64.00	
		QUANTITY OF 2				
/02/10		LEVOFLOXACIN 250MG UD TAB		77.50-	77.50-	
/02/10		CARVEDILOL 12.5MG UD TAB		49.50	49.50	
		QUANTITY OF 3				
/02/10		GUAIFENESIN 600MG LA UD TAB		8.00	8.00	
		QUANTITY OF 2				
/02/10		HYDROCODONE W/APAP 10/325 UD		8.50	8.50	
/03/10		FUROSEMIDE 40MG UD TAB		4.00	4.00	
/03/10		INSULIN ASPART 100U/ML		308.00	308.00	
/03/10		POLYETHYLENE GLYCOL 17GM UD PKT		16.50	16.50	
/03/10		POTASSIUM CL 20MEQ SR UD TAB		4.50	4.50	
/03/10	J1815	INSULIN HUMAN REGULAR 3ML VIAL		55.00	55.00	
/03/10		DARBEPOETIN 100MCG/0.5ML SYR INJ		1835.00	1835.00	
/03/10		DOCUSATE SODIUM 100MG UD CAP		8.00	8.00	
		QUANTITY OF 2				
/03/10		OXYCODONE 5MG/ACETAMIN 325MG TAB		11.00	11.00	
/03/10		NYSTATIN 100,000U/GM CR 30GM		46.00	46.00	
/03/10		NIFEDIPINE 30MG SR UD TAB		33.00	33.00	
		QUANTITY OF 2				
/03/10		OMEPRAZOLE 20MG SR UD CAP		64.00	64.00	
		QUANTITY OF 2				
/03/10		MULTIVITAMINS UD		8.00	8.00	
		QUANTITY OF 2				
/03/10		FERROUS FUM W/DOCUSATE NA UD CAP		8.00	8.00	
		QUANTITY OF 2				
/03/10		CARVEDILOL 12.5MG UD TAB		49.50	49.50	
		QUANTITY OF 3				
/03/10		GUAIFENESIN 600MG LA UD TAB		8.00	8.00	
		QUANTITY OF 2				
/03/10		HYDROCODONE W/APAP 10/325 UD		17.00	17.00	
		QUANTITY OF 2				
/04/10		WARFARIN 2MG UD TAB		7.00	7.00	
/04/10		POLYETHYLENE GLYCOL 17GM UD PKT		16.50	16.50	
/04/10		DOCUSATE SODIUM 100MG UD CAP		8.00	8.00	
		QUANTITY OF 2				
/04/10		OXYCODONE 5MG/ACETAMIN 325MG TAB		44.00	44.00	
		QUANTITY OF 4				
/04/10		NIFEDIPINE 30MG SR UD TAB		33.00	33.00	
		QUANTITY OF 2				
/04/10		OMEPRAZOLE 20MG SR UD CAP		64.00	64.00	
		QUANTITY OF 2				
/04/10		MULTIVITAMINS UD		4.00	4.00	
/04/10		FERROUS FUM W/DOCUSATE NA UD CAP		4.00	4.00	

Fees for physician services, consultations and interpretations are billed individually and are not included as part of the hospital invoice.

63984C

		Insurance portion computed from information verified by employer or insurance carrier and may be subject to change	
	02/21/11		4

/04/10	CARVEDILOL 12.5MG UD TAB	49.50	49.50
	QUANTITY OF 3		
/04/10	GUAIFENESIN 600MG LA UD TAB	8.00	8.00
	QUANTITY OF 2		
/05/10	WARDARIN 2.5MG UD TAB	7.50	7.50
/05/10	POLYETHYLENE GLYCOL 17GM UD PKT	16.50	16.50
/05/10	DARBEPOETIN 100MCG/0.5ML SYR INJ	1835.00	1835.00
/05/10	DOCUSATE SODIUM 100MG UD CAP	8.00	8.00
	QUANTITY OF 2		
/05/10	OXYCODONE 5MG/ACETAMIN 325MG TAB	33.00	33.00
	QUANTITY OF 3		
/05/10	NIFEDIPINE 30MG SR UD TAB	33.00	33.00
	QUANTITY OF 2		
/05/10	OMEPRAZOLE 20MG SR UD CAP	64.00	64.00
	QUANTITY OF 2		
/05/10	MULTIVITAMINS UD	4.00	4.00
/05/10	FERROUS FUM W/DOCUSATE NA UD CAP	4.00	4.00
/05/10	CARVEDILOL 12.5MG UD TAB	33.00	33.00
	QUANTITY OF 2		
/05/10	GUAIFENESIN 600MG LA UD TAB	8.00	8.00
	QUANTITY OF 2		
/06/10	WARDARIN 2.5MG UD TAB	7.50	7.50
/06/10	ZOLPIDEM 5MG UD TAB	23.50	23.50
/06/10	POLYETHYLENE GLYCOL 17GM UD PKT	16.50	16.50
/06/10	DOCUSATE SODIUM 100MG UD CAP	8.00	8.00
	QUANTITY OF 2		
/06/10	OXYCODONE 5MG/ACETAMIN 325MG TAB	44.00	44.00
	QUANTITY OF 4		
/06/10	NIFEDIPINE 30MG SR UD TAB	33.00	33.00
	QUANTITY OF 2		
/06/10	OMEPRAZOLE 20MG SR UD CAP	64.00	64.00
	QUANTITY OF 2		
/06/10	MULTIVITAMINS UD	4.00	4.00
/06/10	FERROUS FUM W/DOCUSATE NA UD CAP	4.00	4.00
/06/10	CARVEDILOL 12.5MG UD TAB	33.00	33.00
	QUANTITY OF 2		
/06/10	GUAIFENESIN 600MG LA UD TAB	8.00	8.00
	QUANTITY OF 2		
/07/10	WARDARIN 2.5MG UD TAB	7.50	7.50
/07/10	POLYETHYLENE GLYCOL 17GM UD PKT	16.50	16.50
/07/10	KENADERM 60GM OINTMENT	294.00	294.00
/07/10	DOCUSATE SODIUM 100MG UD CAP	8.00	8.00
	QUANTITY OF 2		
/07/10	OXYCODONE 5MG/ACETAMIN 325MG TAB	33.00	33.00
	QUANTITY OF 3		
/07/10	NIFEDIPINE 30MG SR UD TAB	33.00	33.00
	QUANTITY OF 2		
/07/10	OMEPRAZOLE 20MG SR UD CAP	64.00	64.00
	QUANTITY OF 2		
/07/10	MULTIVITAMINS UD	4.00	4.00
/07/10	FERROUS FUM W/DOCUSATE NA UD CAP	4.00	4.00
/07/10	CARVEDILOL 12.5MG UD TAB	33.00	33.00
	QUANTITY OF 2		

Fees for physician services, consultations and interpretations are billed individually and are not included as part of the hospital invoice.

Date	Code	Description		
11/07/10		GUAIFENESIN 600MG LA UD TAB	8.00	8.00
		QUANTITY OF 2		
11/08/10		POLYETHYLENE GLYCOL 17GM UD PKT	16.50	16.50
11/08/10		OXYCODONE 5MG/ACETAMIN 325MG TAB	22.00	22.00
		QUANTITY OF 2		
11/08/10		OMEPRAZOLE 20MG SR UD CAP	64.00	64.00
		QUANTITY OF 2		
11/08/10		FERROUS FUM W/DOCUSATE NA UD CAP	4.00	4.00
11/08/10		CARVEDILOL 12.5MG UD TAB	33.00	33.00
		QUANTITY OF 2		
	TOTAL	PHARMACY	9150.50	9150.50
10/29/10	85730	THROMBOPLASTIN TIME PART PTT	148.00	148.00
10/29/10	85610	PROTHROMBIN TIME PT	237.00	237.00
		QUANTITY OF 2		
10/29/10	85027	COMPLETE BLOOD COUNT CBC	116.00	116.00
10/29/10	80048	BASIC METABOLIC PANEL TOTAL CALCIUM	302.50	302.50
10/29/10	81001	URINALYSIS CHEMICAL & MICRO	130.50	130.50
10/30/10	85610	PROTHROMBIN TIME PT	118.50	118.50
10/30/10	87040	BLOOD CULTURE AEROBIC & ANAEROBIC	655.00	655.00
		QUANTITY OF 2		
10/31/10	85007	MANUAL DIFFERENTIAL	29.50	29.50
10/31/10	85610	PROTHROMBIN TIME PT	118.50	118.50
10/31/10	85027	COMPLETE BLOOD COUNT CBC	116.00	116.00
10/31/10	83735	MAGNESIUM	140.50	140.50
10/31/10	80048	BASIC METABOLIC PANEL TOTAL CALCIUM	302.50	302.50
11/01/10	85610	PROTHROMBIN TIME PT	118.50	118.50
11/02/10	85610	PROTHROMBIN TIME PT	118.50	118.50
11/03/10	85025	COMPLETE BLD COUNT W/AUTO DIFF	133.00	133.00
11/03/10	85610	PROTHROMBIN TIME PT	118.50	118.50
11/03/10	80048	BASIC METABOLIC PANEL TOTAL CALCIUM	302.50	302.50
11/03/10	81001	URINALYSIS CHEMICAL & MICRO	130.50	130.50
11/04/10	85025	COMPLETE BLD COUNT W/AUTO DIFF	133.00	133.00
11/04/10	85610	PROTHROMBIN TIME PT	118.50	118.50
11/04/10	83735	MAGNESIUM	140.50	140.50
11/04/10	80048	BASIC METABOLIC PANEL TOTAL CALCIUM	302.50	302.50
11/05/10	85610	PROTHROMBIN TIME PT	118.50	118.50
11/06/10	85025	COMPLETE BLD COUNT W/AUTO DIFF	133.00	133.00
11/06/10	85610	PROTHROMBIN TIME PT	118.50	118.50
11/06/10	80048	BASIC METABOLIC PANEL TOTAL CALCIUM	302.50	302.50
11/07/10	85610	PROTHROMBIN TIME PT	118.50	118.50
11/08/10	85025	COMPLETE BLD COUNT W/AUTO DIFF	133.00	133.00
11/08/10	85610	PROTHROMBIN TIME PT	118.50	118.50
11/08/10	80048	BASIC METABOLIC PANEL TOTAL CALCIUM	302.50	302.50
	TOTAL	LABORATORY	5375.50	5375.50
10/30/10	71010	PORTABLE CHEST 1 VIEW	329.25	329.25
11/03/10	71010	PORTABLE CHEST 1 VIEW	329.25	329.25
	TOTAL	RADIOLOGY - DIAGNOSTIC	658.50	658.50
10/29/10	97001GP	PT EVALUATION - INTERMEDIATE	341.25	341.25
10/29/10	97530GP	THERAPEUTIC ACT PER 15 MIN-PT	157.50	157.50
10/29/10	97116GP	GAIT TRAINING PER 15 MIN - PT	121.50	121.50

Fees for physician services, consultations and interpretations are billed
individually and are not included as part of the hospital invoice.

K35

			02/21/11	

Insurance portion computed from information verified by employer or insurance carrier and may be subject to change

Page No. 6

1/30/10	97112GP	NEUROMUSCLR RE-ED PT PR 15MINS	359.00	359.00
		QUANTITY OF 2		
1/30/10	97110GP	THERAPEUTIC EXER PER 15MIN-PT	342.00	342.00
		QUANTITY OF 2		
1/30/10	97116GP	GAIT TRAINING PER 15 MIN - PT	243.00	243.00
		QUANTITY OF 2		
1/01/10	97110GP	THERAPEUTIC EXER PER 15MIN-PT	1026.00	1026.00
		QUANTITY OF 6		
1/02/10	97110GP	THERAPEUTIC EXER PER 15MIN-PT	1026.00	1026.00
		QUANTITY OF 6		
1/03/10	97110GP	THERAPEUTIC EXER PER 15MIN-PT	1026.00	1026.00
		QUANTITY OF 6		
1/04/10	97110GP	THERAPEUTIC EXER PER 15MIN-PT	1026.00	1026.00
		QUANTITY OF 6		
1/05/10	97110GP	THERAPEUTIC EXER PER 15MIN-PT	1026.00	1026.00
		QUANTITY OF 6		
1/06/10	97110GP	THERAPEUTIC EXER PER 15MIN-PT	171.00	171.00
1/06/10	97116GP	GAIT TRAINING PER 15 MIN - PT	364.50	364.50
		QUANTITY OF 3		
	TOTAL	PHYSICAL THERAPY	7229.75	7229.75
1/29/10	97003GO	OT EVALUATION - COMPLEX	386.50	386.50
1/30/10	97535GO	SELF-CARE ADL TRAIN PR 15MN-OT	398.00	398.00
		QUANTITY OF 2		
1/30/10	97110GO	THERAPEUTIC EXER PER 15MIN-OT	342.00	342.00
		QUANTITY OF 2		
1/30/10	97530GO	THERAPEUTIC ACT PER 15 MIN-OT	315.00	315.00
		QUANTITY OF 2		
1/01/10	97535GO	SELF-CARE ADL TRAIN PR 15MN-OT	199.00	199.00
1/01/10	97110GO	THERAPEUTIC EXER PER 15MIN-OT	342.00	342.00
		QUANTITY OF 2		
1/01/10	97530GO	THERAPEUTIC ACT PER 15 MIN-OT	472.50	472.50
		QUANTITY OF 3		
1/02/10	97535GO	SELF-CARE ADL TRAIN PR 15MN-OT	796.00	796.00
		QUANTITY OF 4		
1/02/10	97110GO	THERAPEUTIC EXER PER 15MIN-OT	342.00	342.00
		QUANTITY OF 2		
1/02/10	97530GO	THERAPEUTIC ACT PER 15 MIN-OT	315.00	315.00
		QUANTITY OF 2		
1/03/10	97535GO	SELF-CARE ADL TRAIN PR 15MN-OT	398.00	398.00
		QUANTITY OF 2		
1/03/10	97530GO	THERAPEUTIC ACT PER 15 MIN-OT	630.00	630.00
		QUANTITY OF 4		
1/04/10	97530GO	THERAPEUTIC ACT PER 15 MIN-OT	945.00	945.00
		QUANTITY OF 6		
1/05/10	97535GO	SELF-CARE ADL TRAIN PR 15MN-OT	199.00	199.00
1/05/10	97530GO	THERAPEUTIC ACT PER 15 MIN-OT	787.50	787.50
		QUANTITY OF 5		
1/06/10	97535GO	SELF-CARE ADL TRAIN PR 15MN-OT	796.00	796.00
		QUANTITY OF 4		
1/06/10	97530GO	THERAPEUTIC ACT PER 15 MIN-OT	315.00	315.00
		QUANTITY OF 2		
	TOTAL	OCCUPATIONAL THERAPY	7978.50	7978.50

Fees for physician services, consultations and interpretations are billed individually and are not included as part of the hospital invoice.

63550

				Statement Date	Insurance portion removed from information received by employee or insurance carrier and may be subject to change.	Page No.
				02/21/11		7

Date		Description		Charges		
1/02/10		TR EVALUATION		197.25	197.25	
	TOTAL	OTHER THERAPEUTIC SERVICE		197.25	197.25	
			TOTAL CHARGES	43053.00	43053.00	.00
1/17/10	07003700	GOVERNMENTAL PAYOR DISCOUNT			31819.25-	
2/02/10	00286328	PAYMENT			22016.03-	
2/02/10	07003700	GOVERNMENTAL PAYOR DISCOUNT			31819.25	
2/02/10	07003700	GOVERNMENTAL PAYOR DISCOUNT			19793.97-	
2/09/10	00288944	PAYMENT				
2/16/10	00287797	PAYMENT				3431.45-
2/21/11	07006257	ADMIN DEC PRIVATE ROOM				1243.00-
		TOTAL PAYMENTS AND ADJUSTMENTS			41810.00-	4674.45-
			ADJUSTED TOTAL	3431.45-	1243.00	.00
			PRIOR BALANCE			.00
			NO PAYMENT DUE			4674.45-

Fees for physician services, consultations and interpretations are billed individually and are not included as part of the hospital invoice.

K355

Patient Statement of Account

system

02/21/11

Insurance portion computed
from information verified
by employer or insurance
carrier and may be subject
to change.

Page No.
1

------- DETAIL CHARGES -------

'20/10		PRIVATE - ROOM/BOARD 0773A	1133.00	1133.00
'21/10		PRIVATE - ROOM/BOARD 0772A	1133.00	1133.00
'22/10		PRIVATE - ROOM/BOARD 0772A	1133.00	1133.00
'23/10		PRIVATE - ROOM/BOARD 0772A	1133.00	1133.00
'24/10		PRIVATE - ROOM/BOARD 0772A	1133.00	1133.00
'25/10		PRIVATE - ROOM/BOARD 0772A	1133.00	1133.00
'26/10		PRIVATE - ROOM/BOARD 0772A	1133.00	1133.00
'27/10		PRIVATE - ROOM/BOARD 0772A	1133.00	1133.00
	TOTAL	PRIVATE - ROOM/BOARD	9064.00	9064.00
'20/10	J0295	AMPICILLIN/SULBACTAM 1.5GM ADV	90.50	90.50
'20/10	J0360	HYDRALAZINE 20MG/ML INJ	322.00	322.00
		QUANTITY OF 4		
'20/10	J7030	IV-SODIUM CHLORIDE 0.9% 1000ML	115.50	115.50
		QUANTITY OF 3		
'20/10		FLUTICASONE 50MCG NASAL SPR	356.00	356.00
'20/10		NACI 0.65% NOSE SPRAY 45ML	16.50	16.50
'20/10	J1815	INSULIN HUMAN REGULAR 3ML VIAL	55.00	55.00
'20/10		IV-1/2 NS 50ML ADV	49.50	49.50
'20/10		OMEPRAZOLE 20MG SR UD CAP	128.00	128.00
		QUANTITY OF 4		
'20/10		INSULIN HUMAN NPHREG 70/30UML VL	66.00	66.00
'20/10	Q0179	ONDANSETRON 4MG UD TAB	540.00	540.00
		QUANTITY OF 4		
'20/10		CARVEDILOL 12.5MG UD TAB	16.50	16.50
'20/10		GUAIFENESIN 600MG LA UD TAB	4.00	4.00
'21/10	J0295	AMPICILLIN/SULBACTAM 1.5GM ADV	90.50	90.50
'21/10	J3370	VANCOMYCIN 500MG INJ	75.00	75.00
		QUANTITY OF 2		
'21/10	J7030	IV-SODIUM CHLORIDE 0.9% 1000ML	77.00	77.00
		QUANTITY OF 2		
'21/10	J1815	INSULIN GLARGINE 100UNIT/ML PEN	444.00	444.00
		QUANTITY OF 2		
'21/10		HYDROCODONE W/APAP 5/325MG UD	18.00	18.00
		QUANTITY OF 4		
'21/10		SODIUM POLYSTYRENE SULF. 15GM/60ML(60ML)	268.00	268.00
		QUANTITY OF 4		
'21/10	J7050	IV-SOD CHLOR 0.9% 50ML MB-PLUS	271.50	271.50
'21/10	J1815	INSULIN HUMAN REGULAR 3ML VIAL	110.00	110.00
		QUANTITY OF 2		
'21/10	J0692	CEFEPIME 1GM VIAL	154.50	154.50
'21/10	J1650	ENOXAPARIN 30MG INJ	154.50	154.50
'21/10		IV-1/2 NS 50ML ADV	49.50	49.50
'21/10	J7050	IV-1/2 NS 250ML	36.00	36.00
'21/10		DOCUSATE SODIUM 100MG UD CAP	8.00	8.00
		QUANTITY OF 2		
'21/10		NIFEDIPINE 30MG SR UD TAB	33.00	33.00
		QUANTITY OF 2		
'21/10		OMEPRAZOLE 20MG SR UD CAP	64.00	64.00
		QUANTITY OF 2		

Fees for physician services, consultations and interpretations are billed
individually and are not included as part of the hospital invoice.

Date	Code	Description	Amount	Amount
10/21/10		CARVEDILOL 12.5MG UD TAB	33.00	33.00
10/21/10		QUANTITY OF 2		
10/21/10		GUAIFENESIN 600MG LA UD TAB	8.00	8.00
		QUANTITY OF 2		
10/21/10		VALSARTAN 160MG UD TAB	34.00	34.00
		QUANTITY OF 2		
10/22/10		OPH LUBRICANT OINT 3.5 GM	29.50	29.50
10/22/10	J3010	FENTANYL CITRATE 50MCG/ML AMP 5ML	32.50	32.50
10/22/10		VECURONIUM 2MG/ML AMP 5ML	94.50	94.50
10/22/10		STERILE H2O INJ 10ML AMP (ES)	9.00	9.00
10/22/10		CEFAZOLIN 1GM ADV VL	26.00	26.00
10/22/10		MORPHINE SO4 1MG/ML VL 30ML	97.00	97.00
10/22/10		CEFAZOLIN 1GM INJ	114.00	114.00
		QUANTITY OF 4		
10/22/10		ROCURONIUM 50MG INJ	128.50	128.50
10/22/10	J2710	NEOSTIGMINE 0.5MG/ML VL 10ML	47.50	47.50
10/22/10		BACITRACIN 50,000U INJ (UJ)	153.00	153.00
10/22/10	J3370	VANCOMYCIN 500MG INJ	150.00	150.00
		QUANTITY OF 4		
10/22/10	J7030	IV-SODIUM CHLORIDE 0.9% 1000ML	115.50	115.50
		QUANTITY OF 3		
10/22/10	J7120	IV-LACTATED RINGER'S 1000ML SOLN.	36.50	36.50
10/22/10	J1815	INSULIN GLARGINE 100UNIT/ML PEN	222.00	222.00
10/22/10		HYDROCODONE W/APAP 5/325MG UD	9.00	9.00
		QUANTITY OF 2		
10/22/10		SOL IRRG SOD CHL 1000CC	13.50	13.50
10/22/10		GLYCOPYRROLATE 0.2MG/ML VL 1ML	27.00	27.00
		QUANTITY OF 3		
10/22/10	J3010	FENTANYL CITRATE 50MCG/ML INJ 2ML	9.00	9.00
10/22/10	J1940	FUROSEMIDE 10MG/ML INJ 2ML	9.00	9.00
10/22/10	J7050	IV-SOD CHLOR 0.9% 50ML MB-PLUS	543.00	543.00
		QUANTITY OF 2		
10/22/10		EPHEDRINE SO4 50MG/ML INJ 1ML	9.00	9.00
10/22/10		PROPOFOL 10MG/ML AMP 20ML	117.50	117.50
10/22/10	J0692	CEFEPIME-ION VIAL	309.00	309.00
		QUANTITY OF 2		
10/22/10	J1170	HYDROMORPHONE 2MG/ML INJ 1ML SYG	10.00	10.00
10/22/10		SODIUM CHLORIDE 0.9% INJ. 20ML	9.00	9.00
10/22/10		LIDOCAINE 1% SD VL 2ML ANE	20.50	20.50
10/22/10		LIDOCAINE 2% VL 5ML ANE	28.00	28.00
10/22/10	J2250	MIDAZOLAM 1MG/ML 5ML	18.00	18.00
10/22/10	J2405	ONDANSETRON 4MG INJ	160.50	160.50
10/22/10		NOREPINEPHRINE 200MCG INJ	101.00	101.00
10/22/10		IV-1/2 NS 50ML ADV	49.50	49.50
10/22/10	J7050	IV-1/2 NS 250ML	72.00	72.00
		QUANTITY OF 2		
10/22/10		DOCUSATE SODIUM 100MG UD CAP	4.00	4.00
10/22/10		NIFEDIPINE 30MG SR UD TAB	16.50	16.50
10/22/10		OMEPRAZOLE 20MG SR UD CAP	64.00	64.00
		QUANTITY OF 2		
10/22/10		CARVEDILOL 12.5MG UD TAB	33.00	33.00
		QUANTITY OF 2		
10/22/10		GUAIFENESIN 600MG LA UD TAB	4.00	4.00

Fees for physician services, consultations and interpretations are billed
individually and are not included as part of the hospital invoice.

K355

Insurance portion computed from information verified by employer or insurance carrier and may be subject to charge.

02/21/11

Date	Code	Description	Amount	Amount
0/23/10		CEFAZOLIN 1GM ADV VL	52.00	52.00
		QUANTITY OF 2		
0/23/10		MORPHINE SO4 1MG/ML VL 30ML	97.00	97.00
0/23/10		DEXTROSE 50% SYG 50ML	39.00	39.00
0/23/10	J3370	VANCOMYCIN 500MG INJ	150.00	150.00
		QUANTITY OF 4		
0/23/10	J7120	IV-LACTATED RINGER'S 1000ML SOLN.	36.50	36.50
0/23/10		FLUTICASONE 50MCG NASAL SPR	356.00	356.00
0/23/10		POLYETHYLENE GLYCOL 17GM UD PKT	16.50	16.50
0/23/10	J7050	IV-SOD CHLOR 0.9% 50ML MB-PLUS	543.00	543.00
		QUANTITY OF 2		
0/23/10	J0692	CEFEPIME 1GM VIAL	309.00	309.00
		QUANTITY OF 2		
0/23/10	J1650	ENOXAPARIN 30MG INJ	463.50	463.50
		QUANTITY OF 3		
0/23/10		IV-1/2 NS 50ML ADV	99.00	99.00
		QUANTITY OF 2		
0/23/10	J7050	IV-1/2 NS 250ML	72.00	72.00
		QUANTITY OF 2		
0/23/10		DOCUSATE SODIUM 100MG UD CAP	8.00	8.00
		QUANTITY OF 2		
0/23/10		NIFEDIPINE 30MG SR UD TAB	33.00	33.00
		QUANTITY OF 2		
0/23/10		OMEPRAZOLE 20MG SR UD CAP	64.00	64.00
		QUANTITY OF 2		
0/23/10		CARVEDILOL 12.5MG UD TAB	33.00	33.00
		QUANTITY OF 2		
0/23/10		GUAIFENESIN 600MG LA UD TAB	8.00	8.00
		QUANTITY OF 2		
0/23/10		HYDROCODONE W/APAP 10/325 UD	17.00	17.00
		QUANTITY OF 2		
0/24/10	J3370	VANCOMYCIN 500MG INJ	150.00	150.00
		QUANTITY OF 4		
0/24/10	J7050	IV-SODIUM CHLORIDE 0.9% 250ML	37.00	37.00
0/24/10	J7030	IV-SODIUM CHLORIDE 0.9% 1000ML	38.50	38.50
0/24/10		HYDROCODONE W/APAP 5/325MG UD	9.00	9.00
		QUANTITY OF 2		
0/24/10		POLYETHYLENE GLYCOL 17GM UD PKT	16.50	16.50
0/24/10	J7050	IV-SOD CHLOR 0.9% 50ML MB-PLUS	543.00	543.00
		QUANTITY OF 2		
0/24/10	J0692	CEFEPIME 1GM VIAL	309.00	309.00
		QUANTITY OF 2		
0/24/10	J1650	ENOXAPARIN 30MG INJ	309.00	309.00
		QUANTITY OF 2		
0/24/10	J7050	IV-1/2 NS 250ML	72.00	72.00
		QUANTITY OF 2		
0/24/10		DOCUSATE SODIUM 100MG UD CAP	4.00	4.00
0/24/10		NIFEDIPINE 30MG SR UD TAB	33.00	33.00
		QUANTITY OF 2		
0/24/10		OMEPRAZOLE 20MG SR UD CAP	64.00	64.00
		QUANTITY OF 2		
0/24/10		CARVEDILOL 12.5MG UD TAB	33.00	33.00
		QUANTITY OF 2		

Fees for physician services, consultations and interpretations are billed individually and are not included as part of the hospital invoice.

Date	Code	Description	Amount	Amount
0/24/10		GUAIFENESIN 600MG LA UD TAB	8.00	8.00
		QUANTITY OF 2		
0/24/10		HYDROCODONE W/APAP 10/325 UD	17.00	17.00
		QUANTITY OF 2		
0/25/10	J3370	VANCOMYCIN 500MG INJ	75.00	75.00
		QUANTITY OF 2		
0/25/10	J7030	IV-SODIUM CHLORIDE 0.9% 1000ML	38.50	38.50
0/25/10	J1940	FUROSEMIDE 10MG/ML INJ 10ML	44.00	44.00
		QUANTITY OF 2		
0/25/10	J7050	IV-SOD CHLOR 0.9% 50ML MB-PLUS	271.50	271.50
0/25/10	J0692	CEFEPIME 1GM VIAL	154.50	154.50
0/25/10	J1650	ENOXAPARIN 30MG INJ	309.00	309.00
		QUANTITY OF 2		
0/25/10	J7050	IV-1/2 NS 250ML	36.00	36.00
0/25/10		DOCUSATE SODIUM 100MG UD CAP	4.00	4.00
0/25/10		NIFEDIPINE 30MG SR UD TAB	33.00	33.00
		QUANTITY OF 2		
0/25/10		OMEPRAZOLE 20MG SR UD CAP	64.00	64.00
		QUANTITY OF 2		
0/25/10		CARVEDILOL 12.5MG UD TAB	33.00	33.00
		QUANTITY OF 2		
0/25/10		GUAIFENESIN 600MG LA UD TAB	8.00	8.00
		QUANTITY OF 2		
0/25/10		HYDROCODONE W/APAP 10/325 UD	17.00	17.00
		QUANTITY OF 2		
0/26/10	J7030	IV-SODIUM CHLORIDE 0.9% 1000ML	38.50	38.50
0/26/10		FUROSEMIDE 40MG UD TAB	4.00	4.00
0/26/10	J1815	INSULIN GLARGINE 100UNIT/ML PEN	222.00	222.00
0/26/10		POTASSIUM Cl 20MEQ SR UD TAB	4.50	4.50
0/26/10	J1815	INSULIN HUMAN REGULAR 3ML VIAL	55.00	55.00
0/26/10	J1650	ENOXAPARIN 30MG INJ	309.00	309.00
		QUANTITY OF 2		
0/26/10		NIFEDIPINE 30MG SR UD TAB	33.00	33.00
		QUANTITY OF 2		
0/26/10		OMEPRAZOLE 20MG SR UD CAP	64.00	64.00
		QUANTITY OF 2		
0/26/10		CARVEDILOL 12.5MG UD TAB	33.00	33.00
		QUANTITY OF 2		
0/26/10		GUAIFENESIN 600MG LA UD TAB	8.00	8.00
		QUANTITY OF 2		
0/26/10		HYDROCODONE W/APAP 10/325 UD	17.00	17.00
		QUANTITY OF 2		
0/27/10		FUROSEMIDE 40MG UD TAB	8.00	8.00
		QUANTITY OF 2		
0/27/10		DIPHENHYDRAMINE 50MG UD CAP	32.00	32.00
		QUANTITY OF 8		
0/27/10		HYDROCODONE W/APAP 5/325MG UD	4.50	4.50
0/27/10		POLYETHYLENE GLYCOL 17GM UD PKT	16.50	16.50
0/27/10		POTASSIUM Cl 20MEQ SR UD TAB	13.50	13.50
		QUANTITY OF 3		
0/27/10	J1650	ENOXAPARIN 30MG INJ	309.00	309.00
		QUANTITY OF 2		
0/27/10	J1650	ENOXAPARIN 100MG INJ	360.00	360.00

Fees for physician services, consultations and interpretations are billed
individually and are not included as part of the hospital invoice.

| | | | 02/21/11 | insurance pursue complied from information verified by employer or insurance carrier and may be subject to change | |

Date	Code	Description	Amount	Amount	
10/27/10		DOCUSATE SODIUM 100MG UD CAP	8.00	8.00	
		QUANTITY OF 2			
10/27/10		NIFEDIPINE 30MG SR UD TAB	33.00	33.00	
		QUANTITY OF 2			
10/27/10		OMEPRAZOLE 20MG SR UD CAP	64.00	64.00	
		QUANTITY OF 2			
10/27/10		POVIDONE IODINE 10% SOL 120ML	10.50	10.50	
10/27/10		GUAIFENESIN 600MG LA UD TAB	8.00	8.00	
		QUANTITY OF 2			
10/27/10		HYDROCODONE W/APAP 10/325 UD	8.50	8.50	
10/28/10		FUROSEMIDE 40MG UD TAB	4.00	4.00	
10/28/10		WARFARIN 7.5MG UD TAB	9.50	9.50	
10/28/10		HYDROCODONE W/APAP 5/325MG UD	9.00	9.00	
		QUANTITY OF 2			
10/28/10		POLYETHYLENE GLYCOL 17GM UD PKT	16.50	16.50	
10/28/10		POTASSIUM Cl 20MEQ SR UD TAB	4.50	4.50	
10/28/10	J1650	ENOXAPARIN 100MG INJ	360.00	360.00	
10/28/10		DOCUSATE SODIUM 100MG UD CAP	4.00	4.00	
10/28/10		OMEPRAZOLE 20MG SR UD CAP	64.00	64.00	
		QUANTITY OF 2			
10/28/10		CARVEDILOL 12.5MG UD TAB	33.00	33.00	
		QUANTITY OF 2			
10/28/10		GUAIFENESIN 600MG LA UD TAB	4.00	4.00	
10/28/10		HYDROCODONE W/APAP 10/325 UD	8.50	8.50	
	TOTAL	PHARMACY	13887.00	13887.00	
10/21/10		BLOOD ADMINISTRATION SET	241.50	241.50	
		QUANTITY OF 3			
10/22/10		BANDAGE COBAN SELF ADHERENT	18.50	18.50	
10/22/10		CUFF VENAFLOW DISPOSABLE	148.00	148.00	
10/22/10	C1769	GUIDEWIRE GAMMA	511.00	511.00	
		QUANTITY OF 2			
10/22/10		DRILL BIT SYNTHES QUICK COUPLING	775.00	775.00	
		QUANTITY OF 2			
10/22/10	C1713	IMP SCREW SKYLINE	1378.00	1378.00	
10/22/10	C1713	IMP SCREW LOCKING TI 5.0X50 STERILE	2174.00	2174.00	
		QUANTITY OF 2			
10/22/10		BANDAGE ACE/DYNA/HONEYCOMB 6IN	24.50	24.50	
10/22/10		STOCKINETTE IMPERVIOUS LG 12"	46.50	46.50	
10/22/10		DRESSING XEROFORM LARGE	8.00	8.00	
10/22/10		STAPLE SURG SS DISPOSABLE	27.00	27.00	
10/22/10	C1713	IMP SCREW TROCHANTERIC FIXATN	3085.00	3085.00	
10/22/10		ESU PENCIL VALLEYLAB	39.50	39.50	
10/22/10	C1713	IMP FIX NAIL CANN TROCH TI	8391.00	8391.00	
10/22/10		ROD REAMING W/BALL TIP 950MM	317.50	317.50	
10/24/10		BLOOD ADMINISTRATION SET	80.50	80.50	
	TOTAL	MED SURG SUPPLIES	17265.50	17265.50	
10/20/10	G0431	DRUG SCREEN SINGLE DRUG CLASS	536.00	536.00	
		QUANTITY OF 8			
10/20/10	82948	GLUCOSE, FINGER STICK	56.50	56.50	
		QUANTITY OF 2			
10/20/10	85025	COMPLETE BLD COUNT W/AUTO DIFF	133.00	133.00	
10/20/10	84520	BLOOD UREA NITROGEN	67.50	67.50	

Fees for physician services, consultations and interpretations are billed
individually and are not included as part of the hospital invoice.

02/21/11   ✓ 6

Date	Code	Description	Charge	Amount
10/20/10	82565	CREATININE	81.75	81.75
10/20/10	82947	GLUCOSE AUTOMATED	58.75	58.75
10/20/10	82310	CALCIUM	88.25	88.25
10/20/10	89050	EOSINOPHIL COUNT (URINE)	94.50	94.50
10/20/10	80051	ELECTROLYTE PANEL	202.50	202.50
10/20/10	81001	URINALYSIS CHEMICAL & MICRO	130.50	130.50
10/20/10	84156	PROTEIN QUANTITATIVE URINE	103.75	103.75
10/20/10	84166	BENCE JONES PROTEIN ELECTROPHO	324.25	324.25
10/21/10	82306	VITAMIN D 25-HYDROXY	41.60	41.60
10/21/10	83036	HEMOGLOBIN A1C	327.00	327.00
		QUANTITY OF 2		
10/21/10	85025	COMPLETE BLD COUNT W/AUTO DIFF	133.00	133.00
10/21/10	85730	THROMBOPLASTIN TIME PART PTT	148.00	148.00
10/21/10	85610	PROTHROMBIN TIME PT	118.50	118.50
10/21/10	86901	BLOOD TYPING R H FACTOR	77.75	77.75
10/21/10	86886	COOMBS INDIRECT	184.00	184.00
10/21/10	86880	COOMBS DIRECT	80.00	80.00
10/21/10	80048	BASIC METABOLIC PANEL TOTAL CALCIUM	302.50	302.50
10/21/10	80061	LIPID PANEL	224.00	224.00
10/21/10	87040	BLOOD CULTURE AEROBIC & ANAEROBIC	327.50	327.50
10/21/10	86923	CROSSMATCH ELECTRONIC	224.25	224.25
		QUANTITY OF 3		
10/21/10	86900	BLOOD TYPING ABO	92.50	92.50
10/21/10	83970	PARATHYROID HORMONE INTACT	525.25	525.25
10/22/10	85018	HEMOGLOBIN HGB	69.50	69.50
10/22/10	85014	HEMATOCRIT	52.50	52.50
10/22/10	85049	PLATELET COUNT	79.50	79.50
10/22/10	85025	COMPLETE BLD COUNT W/AUTO DIFF	133.00	133.00
10/22/10	83010	HAPTOGLOBIN	272.75	272.75
10/22/10	84100	PHOSPHORUS	102.00	102.00
10/22/10	83735	MAGNESIUM	140.50	140.50
10/22/10	84155	PROTEIN TOTAL	130.00	130.00
10/22/10	84165	PROTEIN ELECTROPHORESIS SERUM	253.00	253.00
10/22/10	83540	IRON	115.75	115.75
10/22/10	80048	BASIC METABOLIC PANEL TOTAL CALCIUM	302.50	302.50
10/22/10	82728	FERRITIN ASSAY SERUM	216.25	216.25
10/22/10	87230	CLOSTRIDIUM DIFFIC TXN ASSAY	248.00	248.00
10/22/10	80061	LIPID PANEL	224.00	224.00
10/22/10	83550	IRON BINDING CAPACITY	133.50	133.50
10/22/10	86923	CROSSMATCH ELECTRONIC	149.50	149.50
		QUANTITY OF 2		
10/23/10	85730	THROMBOPLASTIN TIME PART PTT	148.00	148.00
10/23/10	85610	PROTHROMBIN TIME PT	118.50	118.50
10/23/10	85027	COMPLETE BLOOD COUNT CBC	116.00	116.00
10/23/10	84100	PHOSPHORUS	102.00	102.00
10/23/10	83735	MAGNESIUM	140.50	140.50
10/23/10	80048	BASIC METABOLIC PANEL TOTAL CALCIUM	302.50	302.50
10/24/10	85027	COMPLETE BLOOD COUNT CBC	116.00	116.00
10/24/10	80048	BASIC METABOLIC PANEL TOTAL CALCIUM	302.50	302.50
10/24/10	86923	CROSSMATCH ELECTRONIC	74.75	74.75
10/25/10	85027	COMPLETE BLOOD COUNT CBC	116.00	116.00
10/25/10	89050	EOSINOPHIL COUNT (URINE)	94.50	94.50
10/25/10	83735	MAGNESIUM	140.50	140.50
10/25/10	80048	BASIC METABOLIC PANEL TOTAL CALCIUM	302.50	302.50

Fees for physician services, consultations and interpretations are billed
individually and are not included as part of the hospital invoice.

Date	Code	Description	Amount	Amount
				02/21/11

Insurance portion computed from information verified by employer or insurance carrier and may be subject to change.

Date	Code	Description		
0/25/10	81001	URINALYSIS CHEMICAL & MICRO	130.50	130.50
0/25/10	82570	CREATININE URINE	96.00	96.00
0/25/10	84156	PROTEIN QUANTITATIVE URINE	103.75	103.75
0/26/10	85007	MANUAL DIFFERENTIAL	29.50	29.50
0/26/10	85651	SEDIMENTATION RATE ESR	63.00	63.00
0/26/10	85730	THROMBOPLASTIN TIME PART PTT	148.00	148.00
0/26/10	85610	PROTHROMBIN TIME PT	118.50	118.50
0/26/10	85027	COMPLETE BLOOD COUNT CBC	116.00	116.00
0/26/10	80048	BASIC METABOLIC PANEL TOTAL CALCIUM	302.50	302.50
0/27/10	85027	COMPLETE BLOOD COUNT CBC	116.00	116.00
0/27/10	80048	BASIC METABOLIC PANEL TOTAL CALCIUM	302.50	302.50
0/28/10	85007	MANUAL DIFFERENTIAL	29.50	29.50
0/28/10	85610	PROTHROMBIN TIME PT	118.50	118.50
0/28/10	85027	COMPLETE BLOOD COUNT CBC	116.00	116.00
0/28/10	80048	BASIC METABOLIC PANEL TOTAL CALCIUM	302.50	302.50
	TOTAL	LABORATORY	11472.35	11472.35
0/20/10	71010	CHEST (1 VIEW)	329.25	329.25
0/20/10	73550	FEMUR (2 VIEWS)	444.75	444.75
0/20/10	72170	PELVIS	341.50	341.50
0/22/10	76001	OR EXTREMITY OVER 1 HOUR	1069.00	1069.00
0/25/10	71010	PORTABLE CHEST 1 VIEW	329.25	329.25
	TOTAL	RADIOLOGY - DIAGNOSTIC	2513.75	2513.75
0/20/10	74150	CT ABDOMEN WO CONTRAST	2899.00	2899.00
0/20/10	72192	CT PELVIS WO CONTRAST	2888.00	2888.00
0/20/10	72125	CT CERV SPINE WO CONTRAST	3437.50	3437.50
0/20/10	70450	CT HEAD SCAN ROUTINE	2421.25	2421.25
	TOTAL	CT SCANS	11645.75	11645.75
0/22/10		SURGERY TIME 5 HRS	13254.25	13254.25
	TOTAL	OPERATING ROOM SERVICES	13254.25	13254.25
0/22/10		ANESTHESIA 5.0 HRS	5885.25	5885.25
0/22/10		SUPRANE PER BOTTLE	443.00	443.00
	TOTAL	ANESTHESIA	6328.25	6328.25
0/21/10	P9016	BLOOD BNK PROC-HND LEUK RDC RBC FILTER QUANTITY OF 4	1348.00	1348.00
0/22/10	P9016	BLOOD BNK PROC-HND LEUK RDC RBC FILTER	337.00	337.00
0/24/10	P9016	BLOOD BNK PROC-HND LEUK RDC RBC FILTER	337.00	337.00
	TOTAL	BLOOD PROCESSING & STORAGE	2022.00	2022.00
0/21/10	76770	US RENAL	908.00	908.00
	TOTAL	IMAGING SERVICES	908.00	908.00
0/23/10	97001GP	PT EVALUATION - SIMPLE	292.00	292.00
0/23/10	97112GP	NEUROMUSCLR RE-ED PT PR 15MINS	179.50	179.50
0/23/10	97110GP	THERAPEUTIC EXER PER 15MIN-PT	171.00	171.00
0/24/10	97112GP	NEUROMUSCLR RE-ED PT PR 15MINS	179.50	179.50
0/24/10	97110GP	THERAPEUTIC EXER PER 15MIN-PT	171.00	171.00
0/24/10	97116GP	GAIT TRAINING PER 15 MIN - PT	121.50	121.50
0/25/10	97112GP	NEUROMUSCLR RE-ED PT PR 15MINS	179.50	179.50
0/25/10	97110GP	THERAPEUTIC EXER PER 15MIN-PT	171.00	171.00

Fees for physician services, consultations and interpretations are billed
individually and are not included as part of the hospital invoice.

Insurance portion computed from information verified by employer or insurance carrier and may be subject to change

Date	Code	Description		Charges	Insurance	Patient
10/25/10	97116GP	GAIT TRAINING PER 15 MIN - PT		121.50	121.50	
10/26/10	97112GP	NEUROMUSCLR RE-ED PT PR 15MINS		359.00	359.00	
		QUANTITY OF	2			
10/27/10	97112GP	NEUROMUSCLR RE-ED PT PR 15MINS		538.50	538.50	
		QUANTITY OF	3			
10/28/10	97530GP	THERAPEUTIC ACT PER 15 MIN-PT		630.00	630.00	
		QUANTITY OF	4			
	TOTAL	PHYSICAL THERAPY		3114.00	3114.00	
10/20/10	99284	ER VISIT LEVEL IV		1448.75	1448.75	
10/20/10	51702	CATH URETHRA INDWELLG SIMPLE		650.00	650.00	
10/20/10	96361	IV INFUS HYDRATION EA ADDL HR		1048.00	1048.00	
		QUANTITY OF	2			
10/20/10	96374	INJ IV PUSH SGL OR INITIAL SUB		266.00	266.00	
	TOTAL	EMERGENCY ROOM		3412.75	3412.75	
10/25/10	93306	ECHO 2D W SPEC/COLOR DOP COMP		3729.50	3729.50	
	TOTAL	0483		3729.50	3729.50	
10/22/10		PACU 1.5 TO 2.0 HOURS		1981.25	1981.25	
	TOTAL	POST ANESTHESIA CARE		1981.25	1981.25	
10/20/10	93005	ELECTROCARDIOGRAM		697.00	697.00	
		QUANTITY OF	2			
	TOTAL	EKG/ECG		697.00	697.00	
10/25/10	93970	VENOUS DUPLX SCAN-LOW EXT BILATERAL		1411.00	1411.00	
10/26/10	93971	VENOUS DUPLX SCAN LOW EXT UNI		840.00	840.00	
	TOTAL	PERIPHERAL VASCULAR SERVICES		2251.00	2251.00	
		TOTAL CHARGES		103546.35	103546.35	.00
11/01/10	07003700	GOVERNMENTAL PAYOR DISCOUNT			86116.09-	
11/16/10	00286328	PAYMENT			11827.10-	
11/16/10	07003700	GOVERNMENTAL PAYOR DISCOUNT			86116.09-	
11/16/10	07003700	GOVERNMENTAL PAYOR DISCOUNT			86115.25-	
11/16/10	07003700	GOVERNMENTAL PAYOR DISCOUNT			4383.50-	
11/29/10	00287789	PAYMENT			1100.00-	
12/06/10	07005721	DISC PRG INS PORTION ADJUSTMNT			16.50-	
02/21/11	07006257	ADMIN DEC PRIVATE ROOM				904.00-
		TOTAL PAYMENTS AND ADJUSTMENTS			102642.35-	904.00-
		ADJUSTED TOTAL		0.00	904.00	.00
		PRIOR BALANCE				.00
		NO PAYMENT DUE				904.00-

Fees for physician services, consultations and interpretations are billed individually and are not included as part of the hospital invoice.

K958

			02/21/11	Insurance portion computed from information verified by employer or insurance carrier and may be subject to change.	SM01

----- SUMMARY OF CHARGES -----

-- ROOM BOARD & NURSING SERV --

001	PRIVATE - ROOM/BOARD			
	8 DAYS AT 1133.00	9064.00	9064.00	
	ROOM BOARD & NURSING SERVICES	9064.00	9064.00	.00

----- ANCILLARY CHARGES -----

016	PHARMACY	13887.00	13887.00	
019	MED SURG SUPPLIES	17265.50	17265.50	
026	LABORATORY	11472.35	11472.35	
028	RADIOLOGY - DIAGNOSTIC	2513.75	2513.75	
031	CT SCANS	11645.75	11645.75	
032	OPERATING ROOM SERVICES	13254.25	13254.25	
033	ANESTHESIA	6328.25	6328.25	
035	BLOOD PROCESSING & STORAGE	2022.00	2022.00	
036	IMAGING SERVICES	908.00	908.00	
038	PHYSICAL THERAPY	3114.00	3114.00	
042	EMERGENCY ROOM	3412.75	3412.75	
064	POST ANESTHESIA CARE	1981.25	1981.25	
066	EKG/ECG	697.00	697.00	
088	PERIPHERAL VASCULAR SERVICES	2251.00	2251.00	
151	*** UNKNOWN ***	3729.50	3729.50	
	SUBTOTAL - ANCILLARY CHARGES	94482.35	94482.35	

TOTAL CHARGES		103546.35	103546.35	.00
INSURANCE PAYMENTS RECEIVED		12127.10-	12127.10-	
PATIENT ADJUSTMENTS		904.00-		904.00-
INSURANCE ADJUSTMENTS		90515.25-	90515.25-	
ADJUSTED TOTAL		0.00	904.00	.00
PRIOR BALANCE				.00
NO PAYMENT DUE				904.00-

Fees for physician services, consultations and interpretations are billed individually and are not included as part of the hospital invoice.

K3530

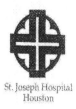

St. Joseph Hospital
Houston

September 13, 1994

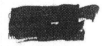

"Our Lord Jesus Christ, suffering in the persons of a multitude of sick and infirm of every kind, seeks relief at your hands."

Dear Doctor ▉

Our routine licensure check with the Texas Board of Medical Examiners (TXBME) has bought the following response regarding an investigation being conducted:

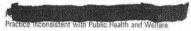

Practice inconsistent with Public Health and Welfare

We are aware that the fact that the Board has received allegations against and/or is conducting an investigation, is in and of itself not a reliable indicator of a possible deficiency. However please submit a complete explanation of the facts, issues and/or cases which led to this investigation. This information will be included in your Quality Assurance file for consideration by the appropriate Section Chief/Department Chairman at the time of your reappointment.

Also, you are required (Article 12.2, Medical Staff Bylaws of St. Joseph Hospital) to report any final adverse action with regard to your license, DEA, DPS registration. This should be reported to the Medical Staff Office within thirty (30) days of the final action taken with regard to the above mentioned investigation.

If you have any questions regarding the above, please do not hesitate to call the Medical Staff Office at 757-7505.

Sincerely,

Bess McCalip, C. M. S. C.
Medical Staff Services

Texas State Board of Medical Examiners

1812 CENTRE CREEK DRIVE, SUITE 300
P.O. BOX 149134
AUSTIN, TEXAS 78714-9134

(512) 834-7728
FAX (512) 834-4597

November 4, 1994

 file.

Dear Doctor ▓▓▓▓▓ ;:

I wish to inform you that the investigation of the
allegation(s) which were previously reported to you has ended
and that we are closing the above referenced file number. We
have concluded that there was no apparent violation of the Medical
Practice Act. This closure is not a disciplinary action taken by
this board against you.

Under certain circumstances, you may be required to inform
others that these allegations against you were lodged with this
board. You may report that the allegation(s) was investigated
and that it was determined that there was no apparent violation
of the Medical Practice Act. You may also use a photocopy of
this letter for that purpose.

The Medical Practice Act specifies that our investigative
file is statutorily confidential, it may not be shared with
you. We are also not allowed to disclose to you the complainant's
identity. Please do not request that additional information be
released to you.

Sincerely,

J E m Shee

INVESTIGATIONS DIVISION

JF/tc

Overview of EMTALA Requirements

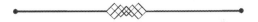

The Emergency Medical Treatment and Active Labor Act (EMTALA) was first signed into law on April 7, 1986, as part of the Consolidated Omnibus Budget Reconciliation Act (COBRA).

1. EMTALA applies to hospitals that participate in the Medicare program and that have an emergency department (ED), and to the physicians practicing in the ED or on-call for the ED.

2. The law protects *all* persons who come into an ED, whether or not they are eligible for Medicare benefits.

3. Every individual requesting emergency services must receive a medical screening examination within the capability of the hospital. The medical screening examination must be sufficient to determine whether the individual has an emergency medical condition.

4. If a patient has an emergency medical condition (which includes a pregnant woman having contractions where there is inadequate time to effect a safe transfer to another hospital before delivery *or* the transfer may pose a threat to the health and safety of the woman or her unborn child), the patient (a) must receive treatment to stabilize the emergency medical condition, or (b) must be transferred appropriately to a facility that can treat the emergency medical condition.

5. The hospital *must* accept the transfer to it of a patient with an unstabilized emergency medical condition *if* (a) the hospital has a specialized capability needed by the patient, (b) the transferring hospital does not have that specialized capability, and (c) the hospital has the capacity (beds, personnel, equipment, physicians on call) to treat the patient.

6. If a hospital believes it received a transfer of a patient in an unstable emergency medical condition, the receiving hospital *must* report this information to CMS or the state survey agency. If a hospital has to transfer a patient because an on-call physician refused to come in, the hospital *must* report the name of that physician to the receiving hospital, which may report the physician to CMS or the state survey agency.

A patient is "dumped" if the patient leaves the hospital at the direction of hospital personnel without being (a) screened according to uniform hospital procedure to determine whether an emergency medical condition exists, (b) stabilized before leaving if hospital personnel discover an emergency medical condition (unless the hospital "appropriately transfers" the patient), or (c) appropriately transferred when the patient has an unstabilized emergency medical condition. The exception to this is when a patient leaves against medical advice (AMA), but the AMA situation must be clearly documented.

A patient is "reverse dumped" if the hospital has a specialized capability needed by a patient with an unstabilized emergency medical condition, the transferring hospital does not have that specialized capability, and the hospital refuses to accept the transfer of the patient even though it has the beds, equipment, personnel, and physicians to treat the patient.

Specifics of EMTALA Requirements

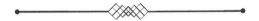

1. The hospital and physician(s) must conduct a sufficient medical screening examination. A patient must receive a sufficient screening examination within the capability of the hospital, including ancillary services routinely available to the emergency department, to determine whether the patient has an emergency medical condition.

   a. An "appropriate screening examination" is one where, with reasonable clinical confidence, the physician can determine whether a medical emergency exists.

   b. The medical screening examination is not an isolated event. The record must reflect continued monitoring until the patient is stabilized or appropriately transferred. There should be evidence of evaluation right before discharge or transfer.

   c. For individuals with psychiatric symptoms, the screening should assess suicide attempts or risk, disorientation, or assaultive behavior that indicates danger to self or others.

2. Under the law, an "emergency medical condition" is as follows:

   a. A medical condition manifesting itself by acute symptoms of sufficient severity (including severe pain, psychiatric disturbances, or symptoms of substance abuse) such that the absence of immediate medical attention could reasonably be expected to result in

      (1) placing the health of the individual (or, with respect to a pregnant woman, the health of the woman or her unborn child) in serious jeopardy,

      (2) serious impairment to bodily functions, or

      (3) serious dysfunction of any bodily part or organ.

      (With respect to a pregnant woman who is having contractions, "serious jeopardy" means that there is inadequate time to effect a safe transfer to another hospital before delivery, or that a transfer may pose a threat to the health or safety of the woman or the unborn child.)

      Caveat: CMS issued a memorandum in early 2002 referring to the rule's definition of "labor" and stating that a woman having contractions is in "true labor" unless a physician certifies that the patient is in "false labor." This memorandum conflicts with the definition of an emergency medical condition as applied to a pregnant woman.

b. A psychiatric patient who poses a threat to self or others.

3. The hospital and physician(s) must not delay the medical screening examination or stabilizing treatment to ask about an individual's method of payment or insurance status. The federal government has issued the following guidelines:

a. The physicians and hospital should not ask about payment or seek prior authorization from a patient's health plan until a patient has received a medical screening examination or has been stabilized. The hospital may obtain prior authorization for services *after* necessary stabilizing treatment is underway.

(1) Medicare and medical managed care plans may not require prior authorization for emergency services and must pay for emergency services without regard to whether the hospital providing the services has a contractual relationship with the plan. (Medicare and Medicaid managed care plans

are required to pay for emergency services based on a "prudent layperson" standard.)

(2) Many states' laws (including those of Texas) apply the "prudent layperson" standard and require health plans to pay for the medical screening examination and necessary stabilizing treatment.

b. The ED physician may contact the patient's physician, including a primary care physician, at any time to seek advice regarding the patient's medical history and needs. *But* if a managed care physician asks that the patient be transferred after being contacted, the hospital and physicians must first meet the EMTALA requirements by concluding the medical screening examination and providing any treatment necessary to stabilize the emergency medical condition before deciding where the patient should go. If the emergency medical condition has not been stabilized, the ED physician may transfer the patient only if (1) the hospital cannot furnish the necessary treatment, and the ED physician certifies that the benefits of transfer outweigh the risks, or (2) the patient requests the transfer.

4. When is a patient stabilized?

   The patient must receive treatment to stabilize the emergency medical condition, which means the hospital and physicians must provide medical treatment as necessary to ensure that, *within reasonable medical probability*, no material deterioration to the condition is likely to result from or occur during a transfer. In the case of a pregnant woman who is having contractions and meets the definition of having an emergency medical condition, the condition is deemed to be stabilized once she delivers the baby and placenta.

5. What is the responsibility of the on-call physicians?

   The ED must maintain a list of physicians who are on call to provide treatment necessary to stabilize an emergency medical condition. An on-call physician must call the ED within a few minutes of being paged and must respond to a request to come to the ED to treat the patient within a reasonable period of time, as determined by the patient's condition and the hospital's policy. (Texas law requires a physician to respond within thirty minutes.)

6. When can a hospital transfer a patient with an *unstabilized* emergency medical condition? *Only if*

    a. the patient or legally responsible person acting on behalf of the patient requests a transfer in writing after being informed of the hospital's obligation to treat patients, *or*

    b. a physician (or other qualified person in consultation with the physician when a physician is not physically present) signs a certification that the "medical benefits reasonably expected from the provision of appropriate medical treatment at another medical facility outweigh the increased risks to the individual's (including the unborn child's) medical condition from effecting the transfer."

7. A transfer of a patient with an unstabilized emergency medical condition must be an "appropriate transfer," which means the following:

    a. The transferring hospital provides medical treatment within its capability and capacity to minimize the risks to health.

    b. The receiving hospital or facility has available space and qualified personnel to treat the patient, has agreed to accept the transfer, and has been provided with the appropriate medical records from the transferring hospital, including copies of

(1) observations of signs or symptoms, preliminary diagnosis, treatment provided, results of any tests;

(2) the informed written consent to transfer *or* the physician certification (or copy thereof); and

(3) the name and address of any on-call physician who has refused or failed to appear within a reasonable time to provide necessary stabilizing treatment.

c. The transfer is made using proper personnel and equipment, as well as necessary and medically appropriate life-support measures. The physician at the *sending* hospital is responsible for determining the appropriate mode, equipment, and attendants for transfer.

8. What about patients who refuse treatment or transfer, and leave against medical advice?

Staff must try to explain the risks and benefits of the examination and treatment, or of the transfer, and get the patient to sign an informed refusal form.

(1) The medical record must describe the examination or treatment refused by the patient.

(2) The informed refusal form must state that the risks and benefits have been explained. If the patient refuses transfer, the reason for refusal should also be documented.

(3) If the patient refuses to sign the written informed refusal form, the hospital must still document the refusal or the circumstances under which the patient left.

9. What is a hospital's obligation to accept the transfer of a patient from another hospital?

A hospital with specialized capabilities or facilities (such as burn units, shock-trauma units, neonatal intensive care units, or, in rural areas, regional referral centers) must accept an appropriate transfer of an individual who requires the specialized capabilities or facilities if the hospital has the capacity to treat the individual (and if the transferring hospital does not have that specialized capability).

Penalties for Physicians Who Violate EMTALA

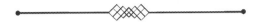

1. Sanctions against physicians

    a. Civil monetary penalties: Any physician who is responsible for the examination, treatment, or transfer of an individual in a hospital (including a physician on call for the care of such an individual) and who *negligently* violates a requirement of EMTALA is subject to a civil monetary penalty of up to $50,000 for each violation.

    b. Exclusion: The Centers for Medicare and Medicaid Services (CMS) can bar a physician from participating in any Medicare program for up to five years if the physician has committed a violation that is deemed "gross and flagrant or repeated."

2. Examples

    a. A physician may be subject to sanctions if he or she

        (1) signs a certification that medical benefits reasonably expected from a transfer to another facility outweigh the risks associated with the transfer, but knows (or should have known) that the benefits do *not* outweigh the risks;

        (2) misrepresents an individual's condition or other information; or

        (3) is on call and fails or refuses to appear to treat the emergency medical condition after the emergency room physician has determined that the patient requires the services of the on-call physician.

    b. The initial examining physician may *not* be subject to sanctions if that physician

        (1) determines that an individual with an emergency medical condition requires the services of a physician listed by the hospital on its list of on-call physicians;

        (2) notifies the on-call physician, who fails or refuses to appear within a reasonable period of time; and

(3) orders the individual's transfer because, without the services of the on-call physician, the benefits of transfer outweigh the risks of transfer.

3. How a physician knows the federal government is considering sanctions

    a. The regional peer review organization (now called a quality improvement organization [QIO]) sends a letter stating that it is reviewing the case and offering the physician the opportunity to discuss the review with the QIO and the opportunity to submit additional information to the QIO before it submits its report to CMS and to the Office of Inspector General.

    b. After the Office of Inspector General receives the QIO's report, it decides whether to impose sanctions. If so, the Office of Inspector General usually sends an informal letter notifying the physician that it is planning to impose sanctions for violations of EMTALA. The letter usually invites the physician to provide additional information and asks the physician to make a settlement offer.

    c. If settlement discussions are not successful, the Office of Inspector General sends a formal notice letter outlining the physician's right to a hearing before an administrative law judge.

d. If, after the hearing, the hospital or physician disagrees with the decision of the administrative law judge, it may appeal the decision to the Departmental Appeals Board. The Departmental Appeals Board has discretion to decide whether to accept the appeal.

e. If the physician disagrees with the decision of the Departmental Appeals Board (or if the Departmental Appeals Board refuses to hear the appeal), the physician may appeal the decision within sixty days to the United States Circuit Court of Appeals in which the hospital is located.

Printed in the United States
By Bookmasters